Praise for *Boost Your Immune Power with Ayurveda*

"Every child is born with innate immunity, but we need to train our bodily cells to fight with certain causative elements in order to boost our immunity."

—Vasant Lad, BAM&S, MASc, Ayurvedic physician and author of
Ayurveda: Science of Self-Healing

T0352960

BOOST YOUR
IMMUNE POWER
··········· WITH ···········
AYURVEDA

About the Author

Janesh Vaidya was born in a family of traditional Ayurveda practitioners in South India. He has spent his life practicing and teaching Ayurveda in India, Europe, and the United States. His health books have sold more than 130,000 copies in Sweden, and have been translated into German, Dutch, Norwegian, Danish, Finnish, and Swedish. Janesh Vaidya lives in Kerala, India. For more information about the author, visit the website JaneshVaidya.com.

BOOST YOUR
IMMUNE POWER
• • • • • • • • • • • WITH • • • • • • • • • • •
AYURVEDA

SIMPLE LIFESTYLE ADJUSTMENTS TO
Balance the Elements in the Body & Mind

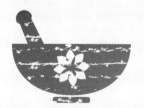

JANESH VAIDYA

Llewellyn Publications • Woodbury, Minnesota

FIRST EDITION
First Printing, 2021

Cover design by Shannon McKuhen
Interior clock illustration on page 33 by the Llewellyn Art Department

Llewellyn Publications is a registered trademark of Llewellyn Worldwide Ltd.

Library of Congress Cataloging-in-Publication Data
Names: Vaidya, Janesh, author.
Title: Boost your immune power with ayurveda : simple lifestyle adjustments
    to balance the elements in the body & mind / by Janesh Vaidya.
Description: First edition. | Woodbury, Minnesota : Llewellyn Worldwide,
    Ltd, [2021] | Summary: "In this book you will discover how to use
    Ayurveda and its branches of food, lifestyle, yoga, and mind development
    to strengthen your immune system through simple lifestyle adjustments"—
    Provided by publisher.
Identifiers: LCCN 2021021230 (print) | LCCN 2021021231 (ebook) | ISBN
    9780738768540 (paperback) | ISBN 9780738768847 (ebook)
Subjects: LCSH: Immune system—Popular works. | Immunity—Nutritional
    aspects—Popular works. | Medicine, Ayurvedic. | Mind and body.
Classification: LCC QR181.7 .V35 2021 (print) | LCC QR181.7 (ebook) | DDC
    616.07/9—dc23
LC record available at https://lccn.loc.gov/2021021230
LC ebook record available at https://lccn.loc.gov/2021021231

Llewellyn Publications
A Division of Llewellyn Worldwide Ltd.
2143 Wooddale Drive
Woodbury, MN 55125-2989
www.llewellyn.com

Printed in the United States of America

Other Books by Janesh Vaidya

For a complete list of books,
visit JaneshVaidya.com/books.

Disclaimer

Dedicated to my grandfather,
who lived and died as a student of Ayurveda

Contents

Charts

INTRODUCTION

The air we breathe, just like the water we drink, is not new. It has passed through countless bodies over millions of years. Since the beginning of life, our planet has been recycling its resources with the support of an ecosystem. However, many of our innovations have destroyed this ecosystem and altered the natural qualities of the water, the air, and the earth we live on. In what we often call the "development" phase of humankind, humans are creating a breeding ground for harmful micro-organisms to grow and spread in the world. Our modern lifestyle is a red carpet inviting these pathogens to invade our organs and generate diseases in our systems.

There are two kinds of diseases that challenge the natural health of a human: infectious and noninfectious. Millions of people have lost their lives in the battle against various infections during several pandemics, and many millions die every year from noninfectious diseases such as cardiovascular disease and cancer or are struggling with severe illness. While plague and cholera were considered the deadliest infectious diseases in past centuries, during the last hundred years the modern world has faced other pandemics, including the Spanish flu, smallpox, tuberculosis, HIV/AIDS, swine flu, and COVID-19.

Although scientists and doctors in our modern medical world are constantly working to keep diseases under control, our current system focuses on treating symptoms and finding quick solutions to switch off the signals from our systems, so the core problems still exist at the base level, popping up to the surface every now and then as different illnesses. If we don't listen to the signals from our body and continue to live our lives going against the laws of nature, polluting the atmosphere and altering the ecosystem of our Mother Earth, then one day, like a boomerang, the results of our actions will return to us with even more vigor.

Before we face an even more dire health situation in our world, let us wake up and work on both of our sides: our inner and our outer nature. While our inner nature is everything inside our skin, including the organs that make up the systems of our body, our outer nature is the body of the earth that contains air, water, and all the living and non-living things on it, including the microorganisms of the ecosystem that we may not even be able to see with our bare eyes.

Considering the fact that our inner body can't function without the support of our outer body, we need to preserve both sides—the nature inside and the nature outside our skin—with equal consideration. For instance, when we cut down a tree, we need to realize that we are mutilating one of our external organs, the lungs of our planet, which convert carbon dioxide into oxygen and are essential to the function of our respiratory system and our life on planet Earth.

Let us draw inspiration from Mahatma Gandhi and create change within ourselves—a shift that will alter the tendencies in the world around us. Let us start the changes, from now on, with the help of the ancient wisdom of Ayurveda.

~Janesh Vaidya

HOW TO USE THIS BOOK

The design of this book gives you the freedom to decide whether you want to move straight into the practical Ayurveda advice or you want to immerse yourself in the theoretical side of this ancient health system. Based on the urgency of the help you currently need for your health, you can plan your reading to make maximum use of this information to improve your health and immunity.

If you already have a basic knowledge of Ayurveda or are in search of a rapid recovery of your immunity and health, you can proceed to chapter 5 to determine your present health status. With the help of two unique self-tests, you can quickly analyze the levels of the presently dominating elements (PDE) in your mind-body system, and use this information to identify your dominant force: kapha, pitta, or vata. Then, using these test results, you can immediately begin to follow the recommendations in this book to design your own individual program based on your dominant force, using the food, lifestyle, meditation, and yoga practices given in the corresponding chapters.

If you are a beginner to Ayurveda or are eager to know more about the principles and the background of this science, I recommend that you read this book from the very beginning and apply the recommendations to your life step-by-step while gradually gaining knowledge through the chapters in the coming pages.

This book has five parts. While part 1 explains the theory and general terms of Ayurveda, parts 2 through 5 focus on the more practical side. Browse through the book and read the opening sections of each chapter to get an idea of what specific information is presented.

Whichever road you choose, during this health journey, your own body and mind are the practice grounds in which you will implement the wisdom of this information. See this reading experience as a voyage, a quest for your ultimate health, and acknowledge the results of your every step toward wellness as an important lesson, leading to utmost health and immunity for the rest of your life.

.... **Part 1** ....
TRADITIONAL KNOWLEDGE
FOR THE MODERN WORLD

My vision is to make Ayurveda accessible to everyone in our modern world, young or old, rich or poor, and, with this ancient health wisdom, to help people grow through the development of their physical, mental, spiritual, and sensuous sides.

Born in a traditional Vaidya family in South India, I was inspired since the early years of my life by my grandma, who took care of the health of the people in her village. That must have been the first spark that later grew in me as the flame of my vision—the vision to support people around the world with my traditional knowledge.

The practice of Ayurveda was recorded in India over five thousand years ago and was the mainstream medical system until the introduction of allopathy and homeopathy during the British colonial times. In ancient India, Ayurveda was practiced professionally by a group of families known as Vaidyas, and the wisdom was passed from one generation to the next, from the eldest Vaidya to the youngest. In those days, every village in India had a Vaidya family taking care of the health of the people in the region. To maintain the healthy regimens of the king and the royal family, the palace appointed a resident Ayurveda physician, who had the noble designation Raja-Vaidya.

However, although Vaidyas are considered to be the godfathers of Ayurveda, with the winds of modernization, many rituals of this

ancient tradition have blown away with time. As one of the last practitioners in the lineage of Vaidyas, my humble desire is to bring the
traditional Ayurveda knowledge to the modern world and spread this
ancient health wisdom among people in all corners of our society
before my tradition sinks into the unknown, just as many other natural
healing practices have disappeared from the world.

I am aware that I have a long way to go to introduce this health wisdom to the over seven billion people in this world, which feels like an
ocean of responsibility. But every morning I wake up with the belief
that every action I take that day will lead me toward my vision, whether
I am caring for the guests at my retreat, giving a lecture in front of a
crowd, meeting a client for a health consultation, or sitting alone in the
silent ambience of my room and writing a book, hoping for this ancient
wisdom to reach an even greater number of people. This belief energizes me during the day, and I go to sleep every night with the same
dream, my vision for this world.

During the last two decades of my travels outside India as an ambassador of Ayurveda, I have learned that I am not alone on this mission.
I have found many like-minded people on other continents, and these
days we are working as a team toward the same mission: to help every
life on this planet achieve maximum health and happiness.

AYURVEDA—LIFE WISDOM FOR OPTIMAL HEALTH

In this chapter I will introduce you to the basic philosophy of Ayurveda and our connection to nature. I will explain how to understand the imbalances in our system and how to correct the root cause of our health problems with the practice of Ayurveda. Before diving deeper into the subject, I will also make sure you are introduced to the Ayurvedic terminology right from the start of your reading experience. For more clarity, I have included the most asked questions about Ayurveda and my answers to them at the end of the chapter.

· · · · · · · · · · · · ·

According to Ayurveda, the richness of your life is not measured by the material possessions and wealth you accumulate during your lifetime, but by your physical health and mental happiness. A rich life will be in tune with nature and constantly cleanse, heal, and protect the body and mind from disease, which helps to maintain a healthy and complete lifestyle. Since Ayurveda is the natural practice of life, any practice that goes against the laws of nature is considered unhealthy living. Unfortunately, our modern society is deviating from natural practices, which is one of the major causes of increasing health problems in recent times.

Sanskrit is one of the most ancient languages in the world, and much of the vital literature about wellness, including the fundamental teachings of Ayurveda, has been documented and passed down through generations in this oldest of Indo-Aryan languages. In Sanskrit, *ayur* means "life" and *veda* means "wisdom," an essential life knowledge for every human to maintain a rich life with maximum immune power and vitality.

The information in this book emphasizes how we can take the knowledge and wisdom of Ayurveda from the Indian tradition and implement it in our modern world without being intimidated by its natural lifestyle and food culture. Other species on our planet follow a natural lifestyle by living in harmony with nature and the seasons. They eat, move, sleep, relax, and make love according to their instincts, while we humans do everything according to the external forces of modern life, which causes major health problems in the body and mind.

In today's world, we compromise our health by adopting a fast-food culture and designing stressful living environments, which weaken the immune system and the body's healing power. Our present comforts and facilities restrict the movement of our muscles and joints and cause poor posture of the spine and shoulders, making us crippled even in our youth. We compromise our personal development and essential sleep for work and nightlife, and we seldom listen to our heart and spend quality time with our loved ones. And still we consider all these changes in our lives as the "developed" phase of humanity.

Regardless of which state we are in right now, with the help of Ayurveda, we have the chance to return to Mother Nature and improve our natural resistance against disease to let the healing begin in our life. Remember that nature has the power not only to decompose but also to regenerate and maintain.

Over time, everything in nature is being composed and decomposed, recycled and repeated, as in day and night, the change of seasons, and birth and death. Apart from us humans, all other species live in harmony with natural law; they don't collect much for the future or carry anything with them for the coming years. In contrast, we humans waste our precious time accumulating possessions and finally leave this wonderful planet without having lived a single day experiencing the miraculous beauty of nature.

The Root Cause of Our Health Problems

The primary reason that Ayurveda has survived throughout the centuries and still stands at the center of our modern civilization is because of its holistic approach to health. This natural science takes care of our physical, mental, and spiritual development during all ages of life and helps us identify the root cause of our physical and mental issues.

Ayurveda considers every pain in the body as a signal and focuses on finding the root cause of the problem, rather than switching off the signals with pills. For instance, if a person suffers from migraines, even though this is a physical symptom, the root cause might be a stressful work situation or a complicated relationship. Even suppressed feelings of grief can cause cellular changes in the body if they are held for a long time, potentially generating harmful tumors.

From these examples, we can understand that a disturbance in our mental system can affect the function of our physical system, and vice versa. And whether it is a long-term physical issue, such as a digestive disorder, or a severe mental issue, such as heavy stress or depression, any disorder in the body or mind will affect the immune system, allowing easy entry for various diseases.

The Five Elements in the Body

The micro level of the body is composed of five elements—earth, water, fire, air, and ether—and our body functions according to the three forces formed by different combinations of these elements. In the terminology of Ayurveda, we call these three forces *kapha* (earth and water), *pitta* (fire and water), and *vata* (air and ether).

When the five fundamental elements in the body are in a state of balance, all our bodily systems—such as the circulatory, respiratory, digestive, urinary, endocrine, lymphatic, nervous, reproductive, skeletal, and muscular systems—function with ease, a sign of perfect health. But if any of the elements gets out of balance, whether through improper diet, lifestyle, or mental practice, it will aggravate the corresponding force and thus create disease in the mind-body system. (We will learn more about the functions of elements and forces in chapter 3.)

The Three Forces and
Their Related Elements

Force	Elemental Combination
Kapha	Earth and water
Pitta	Fire and water
Vata	Air and ether

Fire and Water: The Key Elements of Immunity

Among the five constitutional elements, *agni* (the fire element) controls our immune power through the blood and the circulatory system, protecting the body from harmful microorganisms such as bacteria, viruses, fungi, and parasites. *Jalam* (the water element) and agni (fire) together form the blood and digestive juices and maintain the body's central heating system, which is a key factor in immunity.

In the absence of heat (agni)—in a dead body, for example—the temperature decreases, allowing external microorganisms to enter and decompose the tissues as part of nature's recycling process. Even while we are alive, if our body does not maintain the right amount of agni, harmful microorganisms can defeat our immunity and invade our system, creating dis-ease in the function of our organs.

Immune power varies from person to person and depends not only on which elements are dominant in a person at birth but also the age and season dominating elements. (You will learn more about age and season dominations in the following chapter.) Without knowledge of these natural influences on our body during different stages of our life, if we follow a typical lifestyle, our agni and other elements will become unstable and make the level of immune power fluctuate. Regardless of age and health condition, anyone can rectify the disturbances in their system with personalized food and lifestyle programs and maintain maximum health.

When a person's health is in a state of disorder, one or more elements are out of balance and give off signals in the form of body or mind dysfunction, or both. Neglecting these signals for a period of time weakens the immune system and leads to various kinds of symptoms, and at a later stage can lead to diseases in the corresponding organs. We can recognize these signals even in the early stages by the dysfunction of our body or mind, or both.

If we listen to the signals from our body and mind, we can identify which elements are disturbed in our system. For instance, if we are not eating the right food according to our PDE (presently dominating elements), our digestive system will show signs of the imbalanced elements, such as indigestion (earth-water imbalance), acid reflux (fire-water imbalance), or bloating with gas (air-ether imbalance). Or, if we have a disorder in our mental body, it might manifest as depression (earth-water imbalance), high stress (fire-water imbalance), or anxiety (air-ether imbalance). We will dive deeper into these topics when we learn more about the five fundamental elements and the three vital forces in the coming chapters. But first, let us take a look at the most commonly asked questions about Ayurveda.

Common Questions about Ayurveda

While traveling as an ambassador of Ayurveda, giving lectures and health consultations around the world, I am asked certain questions repeatedly. To get more closely acquainted with this natural health science and its application in your life, here are the most common questions about Ayurveda and my answers.

How Do I Know if I Am in Optimal Health?

Your health is reflected in your immune power, which is controlled by the fire and water elements in your system. A major part of your body's immunity is maintained by the white blood cells in your blood, which search for invading pathogens and fight harmful microorganisms. Any imbalances in the elements, especially in the fire and water elements, directly affect the functions of white blood cells and make the body prone to infection.

You can also analyze your health by checking the state of your digestion, since your digestive tract is the cradle of your immune system and holds the beneficial microorganisms that also fight against pathogens. If you observe these two areas—your blood values and the function of your digestive system—you can determine the status of your immune power and thus the present state of your health. If your blood values are normal and you maintain an excellent metabolism, you can consider it a sign of good immune power—proof of your optimal health.

How Do I Know Whether I Have an Imbalance in My Body or Mind?

Suppose that you are suffering from a deficiency in your blood or an abnormality like anemia. Or perhaps you often experience digestive issues, such as diarrhea, constipation, or gas, or you suffer from fatigue, frequent infections, or colds, or it is taking a long time for a wound in your body to heal. These are all common signs of an imbalanced state of the elements in your body, causing low immunity in the system.

When you notice a sign of uneasiness in your body or mind functions, consider it a disorder—a signal indicating that something is not normal in your health. Be aware of the initial stage of these signals, and address them right away, before they become symptoms and develop into diseases.

Are There Any Quick Remedies in Ayurveda to Balance an Imbalance?

Imagine that there was a fire in your house and the fire alarm was ringing: Would you switch off the alarm or put out the fire? We all know the correct answer, but what are we doing in our modern life in terms of our health? We tend to look for quick fixes to our health problems with temporary solutions and pills.

Whether it is high blood pressure, high cholesterol levels, digestive issues, or other symptoms, there are many easy and fast solutions available in our modern world to switch off the signals of dysfunction. But by depending only on quick-fix pills to shut off these signals, we can never find the root cause and solve the actual health problem. Since every symptom in our body and mind is a signal, we shouldn't switch off these indications with pills or other temporary solutions. Most medications not only affect the organs they are meant to treat, but also have known and unknown side effects that can cause damage to other organs in the body. Treating a symptom only with pills for a long time can collapse the entire system and partially or completely shut off our internal mechanism.

Is Traditional Ayurveda against Modern Medical Practice?

Absolutely not. In our modern society, most people lead a fast-food and fast-paced lifestyle. And because of our unhealthy food habits and unnatural lifestyle, sometimes we need quick solutions to fix our problems. For example, if someone gets in an accident and is fighting for their life, first we need to bring them to the emergency room of a modern hospital. Or if a person leads an unnatural life without listening to the signals from their body or mind and ends up with a life-threatening condition for which surgery might be the only solution, such as a heart attack, then they need the service of medical doctors to save their life.

Can Ayurveda Help with All Kinds of Health Conditions?

Here are the four different health conditions and the use of Ayurveda for each one:

1. *Perfect health:* If your health is perfect at the moment, which means you don't have any imbalances in your body or mind, then you can follow the Ayurveda disciplines as a preventive method to avoid getting any diseases in the coming years.

2. *Getting signals from the organs:* If you notice any signals of dysfunction from your body or mind, you can address the cause of the signals right from the beginning with the natural tools of Ayurveda. In this initial stage of disorder, you typically can balance your elements within a few weeks with disciplined practice and get back to a state of perfect health.

3. *Suffering from symptoms (indicating dysfunction of an organ or an entire system):* If you are already suffering from symptoms and are undergoing medical treatment, start the Ayurveda disciplines as a complementary practice in your daily life to see step-by-step improvements in your health. As you see progress in your health, cut down on the pills you take as your physician advises.

4. *Your health is at risk due to a life-threatening disease:* If your life is currently at risk because of a severe disease, practice Ayurveda as a complementary method to reduce the side effects of any modern medical treatments (such as chemotherapy, which the doctors might need to apply to the body's cells in order to save the person's life, even though it is harmful to healthy cells). In these situations, Ayurveda can help to support a person's system to cleanse and rejuvenate it with the care of nature's essence.

How Do I Use Ayurveda to Boost My Immune Power and Achieve Optimal Health?

By following the natural disciplines of Ayurveda in your daily life, you can balance the levels of the fundamental elements in your system. And once your elements come into a state of balance, your good health will reflect through the resistance power of your body.

As I mentioned earlier, traditional Ayurveda puts an emphasis on finding the root cause of disorders and treating them with natural solutions, rather that suppressing symptoms with temporary solutions. According to this ancient wisdom, you can support your natural state of health by maintaining a discipline in your daily life with three practices: eating the right foods to balance your presently dominating elements (PDE), cultivating and keeping inspiring thoughts in your mind, and maintaining a healthy lifestyle, with sufficient rest and exercise for your present body and mind condition.

You have nothing to lose by trying something new every day. Remind yourself often that nobody ever learned anything thoroughly without making some mistakes. As my grandma used to say, it is better to make a mistake and learn from it than to do nothing. But try not to repeat the same mistakes, as that will reduce your opportunities to try something new or make another mistake. This is one of the basic lessons while you acquire your *ayur-veda*, your life wisdom.

················ **Chapter 2** ·················
AYURVEDA AND IMMUNITY

In this chapter we will look at the primary reasons for low immunity in the human body and its correlation to the three forces: kapha, pitta, and vata. Since our digestive system is the base of our immunity, we will learn about the three different digestive disorders caused by the aggravation of these three forces. We will also examine seven general causes of poor immunity commonly seen in our modern society.

············

One of the major reasons for low immunity and main causes of disease is the accumulation of toxins (*ama*) in the circulatory channels, which blocks the transport of immune cells. If the organs in the digestive system are not functioning well, toxins can accumulate in the channels and disturb the normal function of the entire system, reducing the natural resistance power and vitality of the body. As we learned earlier, agni, the fire element, plays a major role in the function or dysfunction of the digestive and metabolic systems.

In the state of *sama agni* (balanced fire element), the whole process of digestion and metabolism—from the digestion of food and the absorption of nutrients to the distribution, storage, and release of energy at the cellular level, and the elimination of toxins through urine, sweat, and feces—functions without complications. But if the agni in the body is out of balance, three kinds of digestive disorders can occur, which affect the immune power and make the body prone to pathogenic attacks on the organs.

Digestive Disorders That Weaken the Immune System

1. *Manda agni (slow digestion):* Weak digestion results from not having enough agni—the minimum level of digestive fire required for the function of the digestive system. Because of the low level of the fire element in the system, the digestion of food takes more time, creating indigestion and gas-related issues in the stomach. Slow digestion also leads to the accumulation of toxins in the channels, attracting harmful external microorganisms.

2. *Tikshna agni (intense digestion):* This condition is caused by the hyperactivity of agni. With the intense heat of the fire element, the digestive system breaks down the food too fast. In this state of hyperacidic activity, the person is often hungry and dissatisfied even after eating. This condition can cause acid reflux from the stomach and a burning sensation in the esophagus, and if the issue is not addressed in time, it can lead to ulcers.

3. *Vishama agni (difficult digestion):* Erratic digestion is a condition where the digestive system functions unpredictably. In this state, the level of agni can be too high or too low, making the digestion fast or slow. This can create bloating or a burning sensation, or both problems, in the stomach and esophagus. This condition leads to inflammation in the body, which attracts infections and alerts the immune system.

If you are experiencing any of these digestive symptoms, you can conclude that your agni is not in a state of balance at the moment. And since agni is one of the key factors of your immune system, your immune power depends on its stability.

There are several reasons that the agni in your system can get disturbed. Finding the root cause and correcting your digestion and metabolism with a knowledge of Ayurveda is the first step to improve your health.

According to Ayurveda, the three forces (kapha, pitta, and vata) control the overall function of the body, including the digestion and metabolism. While sama agni is the balanced state of the fire element and a controlled state of the three forces in the digestive system, the imbalanced state of the fire element disturbs the forces and causes three kinds of problems in the digestion: disturbed kapha (manda agni), disturbed pitta (tikshna agni), and disturbed vata (vishama agni).

The Correlation Between Agni and Body Weight

Digestion and metabolism play a major role in a person's body weight fluctuations, and there are two kinds of metabolic functions in the body: constructive metabolism and destructive metabolism. Through constructive metabolism, the body receives nutrients from the digested food, generating new tissues and restoring energy in the cells, while through destructive metabolism, energy is released from the cells and the body's excretions are expelled from the system.

Together with jalam (water), agni (fire) forms digestive acids and enzymes that support the breakdown of food in the different stages of digestion, all the way from the tongue to the small intestine. These digestive enzymes can be found in the salivary glands and the pancreas, in the lining of the stomach, and in the small intestine. Among the digestive enhancers, the hydrochloric acid in the stomach contains the highest level of agni.

The enzymes and acids formed by the water and fire elements aid the first stage of digestion and metabolism: to digest the food and absorb the nutrients through the lining of the small intestines, carry them to the cells through the blood, and store them as an energy reservoir or as constructive elements for new tissue.

In the second stage of digestion and metabolism, agni (fire), together with vayu (air), release the stored energy during the body functions and eliminate particles of food waste through the excretory channels.

Each person's level of agni, and thus their digestion and metabolism, changes according to the level of the dominating elements in the body systems. If the earth and water elements dominate the system, the body is driven by the force of kapha, with a tendency to become overweight and have a hard time losing weight because of the gravitational character of this force. But if the air and ether elements dominate the system, the body is driven by the force of vata, and has difficulty gaining and maintaining adequate weight. This person often struggles with low body mass and related symptoms due to the effects of anti-gravity in this force. If the fire and water elements dominate the system, the body is driven by the force of pitta and maintains a consistent weight because of an active digestive system, a steady appetite, and an energetic lifestyle. This helps the metabolic organs in the body receive nutrients in time and eliminate toxins from the channels without interruption. But if pitta is the dominating force in a system, there is also a higher chance of an imbalance in agni, which can aggravate pitta and lead to symptoms and eventually diseases in the digestive organs.

In the coming chapters, you will learn more about these three forces and their effects on the human body in their stable and unstable states.

Seven General Causes of Low Immunity

Before we begin our study of how we can improve our health with the help of Ayurveda, let's look at some general reasons that our immune system may not be functioning at an optimal level.

Though there are many factors that can influence the level of agni in the body and the natural resistance power of our system, there are seven factors commonly seen in our modern society that we should discuss before moving further with our studies.

1. Poor Food Habits

What happens if we fill the tank of a diesel car with gas? It might run for a while, but soon there will be problems with the engine and the car will break down on the road. If we feed our stomach with the wrong food, the wrong fuel, sooner or later our health engine will break down on the road of our life.

Although all cars have similarities in their general function on the road, they are not all the same. Each vehicle differs in mileage and the type of fuel required, in power and performance. Similarly, although we humans resemble one another in our physical features, the shape of our organs, and the general function of our internal systems, we are different in terms of our core nature, our engine. This is why we need to provide the right fuel, the right food, for our digestive system, and not just what can fit in our stomach. But unfortunately we seem to believe that all humans can eat all the foods available at the grocery store.

To correct the function of your digestive system, determine the present state of your digestion and make the modifications needed in your daily food habits accordingly. For instance, if you have less agni in your digestive tract and a bloated stomach with gas or indigestion, then make sure to raise the level of agni by adding enough spices to your food as digestive enhancers. If you have problems with intense fire and are suffering from hyperacidity, heartburn, or acid reflux, then reduce the agni in your system by avoiding strong spices and acidic foods and drinks in your daily diet. (You will find more information and a list of foods that increase and decrease agni in chapters 10 and 11.)

Good health and optimal immunity are reflected in your daily stomach function. If you are a beginner to Ayurveda, gaining the knowledge of this ancient wisdom through reading this book is the first step. I want to remind you to see your body as the primary learning material and to start monitoring the daily function of your stomach, especially after eating each meal. In a healthy state, you have a regular appetite that functions like a clock, and bowel movements will occur one to three times a day, with no constipation, diarrhea, gas, bloating, acid reflux, heartburn, cramps, or other stomach issues. If you have digestion problems, try to change your food habits by adding or eliminating some foods and drinks that you think might be affecting the agni in the digestive tract.

2. Heavy Stress or Depression

Two factors that can reduce the immune power are mental stress and depression. In our modern society, stress is one of the major causes of many health problems. Chronic stress not only affects the function of our metabolism by disturbing the level of agni, but also causes serious damage to the hormonal functions in our endocrine system. For instance, our body has an emergency defense mechanism that releases hormones such as cortisol and adrenaline from the adrenal glands when we are facing a dangerous situation in which the body needs to react fast. When the mind senses an external danger, the pituitary glands in the brain stimulate the adrenal glands to release the hormones that support the body systems to take sudden action.

In an emergency, the cortisol hormones temporarily pause the physical functions of nonessential body systems such as the reproductive and immune systems, and redirect that energy for the fight-or-flight power of the body. Meanwhile, the adrenaline hormones increase the heart rate, boost the blood and oxygen supply, and release glucose, preparing for rapid action of the muscles.

Although cortisol and adrenaline hormones are part of the body's emergency defense mechanism, sometimes non-life-threatening situations can also trigger the adrenal glands. When the mind gets overly excited or stressed, these hormones are released into the blood and prepare the body to act instantly. If we continuously live in stress, our stress hormones, cortisol and adrenaline, will constantly be released into our blood, disturbing the fire element in the body. This pauses the functions of our immune system in order to use the energy to elevate the heart rate and the respiratory and liver functions. If this situation continues for a while, our endocrine system will collapse and our natural resistance power will be weakened by the continuous suppression of our immune system. Heavy stress can also reduce the capacity of our brain to give the right signals to protect our body at times when it needs a defense, like when pathogens are threatening our system.

Other common consequences of living with heightened stress levels are autoimmune disorders. In healthy conditions, our brain senses invading pathogens in our body systems and signals to our immune cells to attack the invader. Our brain is the captain of the army, our immune system, and its orders are vital for victory over our enemies, the pathogens that enter our territory, our body systems. But because of the heavy stress, our brain loses its natural capacity to sense the enemy and to direct our immune system to fight against it. Since the immune system always obeys the orders of the captain, our brain, if it gives a wrong order, our army might even attack our own organs and destroy our own systems. We call this state an autoimmune disease.

Though autoimmune disorders can affect any part of the body, they often disturb the endocrine system, for instance, the natural functions of the thyroid glands and the production of insulin in the pancreas. These disorders also affect the skin (causing, for example, psoriasis), the nerves and muscles (causing multiple sclerosis), the joints (causing rheumatoid arthritis), and the functions of the red blood cells. Auto-immune disorders also increase the risk of certain kinds of cancer and chronic inflammation in the body. The best way to prevent our immune system from entering this state is to provide our brain with enough rest and relaxation by avoiding or reducing stressful situations and thoughts.

With the help of the Ayurveda lifestyle suggestions in this book, you can make necessary modifications in your daily life and save your mind from stress and related symptoms. You can learn more about how to adjust your personal and professional lives with the tools of this ancient health science and avoid stressful situations in your life by maintaining a healthy body and mind.

Another state that weakens the immune system is depression, which is a mental disorder caused by aggravation of the kapha force, driven by the earth and water elements in the system. When a mind is in a state of depression, it slows down the functions of the body systems, including the digestive system and the metabolism. This reduced level of agni not only diminishes the immune power but also causes toxins to accumulate in the channels that block the subtle energies that maintain the overall health and vitality of the person. Because of the blocked channels and increased toxins, the body will be under constant threat from external harmful microorganisms and the diseases they cause.

There are many causes of depression, including medication, drugs, trauma, and grief, which affect us differently according to our prakruti, our birth dominant elements, and any current imbalances in the system. For instance, although grief can develop into depression in anyone's mind, kapha dominant individuals have the biggest risk for this mental issue because of their overattachment to people and to their surroundings. For a kapha dominant, it can be hard to accept that sooner or later everything will change in life, or even disappear.

Since a depressive mind can fall into many unhealthy habits, such as eating disorders and alcoholism, and most people in the world pass through a state of depression at some period in their lives, we have to take this state of mental fall into serious consideration and act in time to overcome it through the disciplined practice of an active Ayurvedic lifestyle, vitalizing food, and energizing exercise.

3. Lack of Rest or Poor Sleep

Is there any better therapy than sleep to restore our energy and maintain good health? From my experience of working with patients, there is no replacement for sleep therapy, and that's why we are supposed to invest around one-third of our life in sleep. During the hours of sleep, our internal systems are cleansed of mental and physical toxins, our old cells are replaced with new ones, and our body and mind are refreshed with vital energies. If we don't get enough sleep, our body won't have enough time to eliminate the toxins, which will then block the circulatory channels and affect the level of agni and thus the immune system. In the long run, the accumulated toxins and fat can create inflammation in the body, low resistance power against infections, and obesity.

Together with the right diet and exercise, quality sleep is a natural rejuvenating therapy. The quality of sleep is measured not only by the total hours of sleep but also by the depth of "total arrest" of our body and mind during those hours. For instance, some people get an adequate number of hours of sleep, but they wake up with tiredness in the body or with a restless mind. This happens when the sleep is shallow and the subconscious mind is awake, though the conscious mind is sleeping. If our mind is concerned with something in our life, such as worries about our own health, our job situation, our relationship with our partner, or anxiety about the lives of close family members, then our subconscious mind can be alert throughout the day and night.

Sleep is a natural rejuvenator of our body and mind systems, and Ayurveda emphasizes giving prime attention to improving the quality of our sleep by understanding the root cause of our sleep problems, redefining our current lifestyle, and learning about the natural sleeping patterns based on the dominating elements in our system. When you understand these two conflicting factors in your life—your mind-body type and the part of your lifestyle that is working against your mind-body type—then you can use the tools of Ayurveda to correct the problem with the right adjustments to your lifestyle and food habits, which will improve the quality of your sleep.

Ojas

Ayurveda describes *ojas* as the tonic of our body and mind, generated and stored in a major part in the region of the heart chakra (center of the chest) during sleep. This subtle energy plays a major role in the overall defense mechanism of the mind-body systems throughout our life. A sufficient amount of ojas in the heart chakra is essential to cleanse, rejuvenate, and protect the systems from disease. When your body lacks sleep, resulting in a deficiency of ojas, you get tired in the body and experience boredom in the mind. A deficiency of ojas in your system can also create pressure in the center of your chest, making it an effort to take full breaths (restricted expansion of the diaphragm). When you are tired, you feel that you want to yawn, but because of the lack of ojas, you can't complete a yawn or take long, deep breaths.

Though many people have sleeping problems, three kinds of sleeping issues are common, which result from imbalances in the elements that dominate the body and mind. For instance, if there is an imbalance in the earth and water elements that aggravates the force of kapha, the person has difficulty waking up in the morning. Even after a long sleep, they wake up with sluggishness in the body and mind. If the elements are in a state of imbalance, pitta dominants (fire and water elements) suffer from light, interrupted sleep, while vata dominants (air and ether elements) struggle to fall asleep. Ayurveda has solutions for insomnia caused by disorders in all the elements, regardless of a person's age and health condition. (We will learn about Ayurveda's solutions for better sleep in chapter 14).

4. Overuse of Pharmaceutical Drugs

Since good sleep is a natural rejuvenator of our mind-body systems and one of the key practices to maintain our immune power and ojas, anything that reduces the quality of our sleep can be considered a destroyer of our immunity and wellness. And the overuse of pharmaceutical drugs plays a big role in disturbing our natural sleep and weakening our body's resistance power.

We know that millions of people in the world are surviving with the support of chemical pills. Our modern society is a fast-food, fast-life, and fast-death culture, and these pills play a major role in keeping us humans alive in modern times. However, some drugs used to treat heart disease and blood pressure variations, for example, can cause sleeping problems. Even an overdose of Ayurveda herbs—ashwagandha, for example—can lead to sleep disorders, since its stimulating effect sometimes disturbs the mind and makes it difficult to get into a deep sleep.

The number of people in the world using drugs such as antibiotics increases every year. The word *anti-biotics* itself means "against life," and we already know that if we use these emergency medications unnecessarily, they can damage the beneficial microorganisms living in our digestive system and create more severe problems in our health. We also need to consider that only a small percentage of the antibiotics produced in the world is used to treat bacterial infections in humans—the rest of the antibiotics produced will reach our bodies indirectly. Enormous amounts of these antibiotics enter human bodies every day through animal products and byproducts, since these antibiotics are used to feed farm animals as a preventive medicine, to treat illness, or for growth promotion. These chemicals enter our body if we consume these animals or their byproducts, such as dairy or eggs, as our food, and the harmful substances are deposited in our metabolic system as toxins that reduce the natural resistance power of the body.

If we choose to continue this food culture, we humans need to prepare for higher dosages of antibiotics every time a new harmful bacterium emerges. Because while our body's resistance power is reduced by the overuse of antibiotics we receive through our daily animal-based food, the bacteria are getting more powerful every year by improving their resistance power against the antibiotics. This is considered a major threat to humans in the near future.

Also remember that beneficial microorganisms, such as the "good" bacteria in our digestive tract, are our primary line of defense against pathogens entering the system. These good bacteria produce "natural antibiotics" to fight against harmful external microorganisms. But the overuse of these drugs, the chemical antibiotics we humans ingest through animal-based food, can collapse the entire defense system lined up in our digestive tract.

5. Use of Alcohol

Most of us already know that socially accepted drugs such as alcoholic drinks reduce the natural vitality of the mind-body system with their slow poisoning effect. Intake of alcohol creates an imbalance in the earth and water elements in the body and disturbs the mucous membrane linings in the respiratory, digestive, and urogenital tracts.

In a healthy body, the earth and water elements maintain the mucous membranes, with their moisturizing property as the first layer of immune cells. Like security guards, these immune cells create a wet surface over the epithelial tissues of the internal channels, where there is a passage of entry or exit for air, water, or food particles. These are the main channels through which most harmful external microorganisms pass into the body. The passages are the eyes, nostrils, mouth, trachea, and lungs, as well as the inner walls of the stomach and the intestines and the channels of the urethra and the vagina.

Continuous use of alcohol damages these protective linings either by draining the moisture content in these cells and defusing their immune power or by generating excess mucus in these channels and creating blockages and inflammation that attract the pathogens. For instance, alcohol can destroy the mucous membranes in the respiratory channels, which allows easy access of infections into the lungs and increases the risk of inflammation in the breathing channels, leading to illnesses like pneumonia and tuberculosis.

Alcohol also creates imbalances in the fire and water elements and affects the function of the digestive system, where the agni, the digestive fire, controls the body's central heating system, the natural maintainer of immune power. With its acidic properties, alcohol kills the beneficial microbes in the intestines that play a major role in fighting against the pathogens. Regular use of these drinks damages the epithelial tissues in the intestines, which makes it more difficult for the blood to absorb nutrients from the food, making the body too weak to maintain a healthy immune system. The damage in the barrier lining of the intestines caused by this liquid form of drug allows the bacteria to pass into the blood and can cause inflammation in the liver.

By disturbing the digestive fire, drugs such as alcohol decrease the level of white blood cells in the blood. (As mentioned earlier, white blood cells are part of the defense system that fights against the pathogens and protects the body from infectious diseases.) Also, alcohol reduces the mobility of white blood cells toward inflammation in the body tissues, where the chances of infection are high and more resistance power is needed.

Intense use of alcohol or other kinds of drugs can collapse the natural state of agni that controls the heating system of the body and make cells cold and prone to external harmful bacteria, virus, fungi, and parasites. An imbalance of the fire and water elements in the body causes destruction of three kinds of cells in our blood: macrophages, T cells, and B cells. While macrophages eat the harmful cells generating in the body, including cancerous cells, T cells function as antibodies against certain pathogens and B cells secrete proteins called cytokines that eliminate the cells affected by harmful microorganisms. When the natural resistance power of these cells is diminished, a major part of our immunity is destroyed in our system. This will allow invading pathogens to enter our body at the micro level.

Heavy drinking can also increase the risk of sexually transmitted diseases, since the resistance power is weaker in the reproductive system when in a state of imbalance in the air and ether elements. On the mind level, the disturbed air and ether elements affect the central nervous system and thus the memory, causing problems such as a lack of concentration, poor coordination of the information assimilated through the senses, and less control of the organs because of the weakening of motor skills.

Though alcohol is harmful for all body types, based on the experiences of my clients, I have seen the worst damage in pitta dominant bodies, where the effects manifest quickly and on a high level. Alcohol has a rapid effect on a pitta-dominated body because the fire element in the body reacts quickly to the similar property in the liquor, like pouring gas on a fire. A vata-dominated body also reacts instantly to alcohol, even in small doses, because of their sensitive central nervous system. On the other hand, the reaction to alcohol is slower in kapha-dominated bodies, and they can hold large quantities. But because of the high capacity of kapha-dominated bodies, they tend to drink larger amounts of alcohol and can become addicted to liquor. And once they are in the habit of drinking, the strong attachment tendencies in their personality make it harder to quit.

6. Destructive Lifestyle

Our lifestyle plays a major role in maintaining our health and resistance power. The lifestyle of an individual is shaped by their living conditions, healthy or unhealthy habits, good or bad personal relationships, professional satisfaction or dissatisfaction, the level of pollution in the atmosphere, climatic conditions, and a close or distant relationship with nature. At any age of life, we can improve our health by making lifestyle adjustments that match our mind-body type. (In the next chapter we will learn about the mind-body type of a human, which is determined by the dominating elements at the time of birth, but can be influenced by age, season, and even the time of the day.)

The immune power differs from person to person, which Ayurveda explains as the resistance power of different body types. For instance, as a general rule, if the body is dominated by the earth and water elements and these elements are in a state of balance, then these types of bodies naturally have high resistance power. But they are also sensitive to damp and are prone to symptoms or diseases in the systems of the upper body, such as the circulatory and respiratory systems.

The fire-water dominant bodies are sensitive to excess heat and often have problems in the digestion-related organs, such as the liver, spleen, pancreas, stomach, and small intestines.

Air-ether dominant bodies are sensitive to cold and are prone to diseases in the lower part of the body, like in the reproductive organs, colon, and rectum.

To achieve maximum health and resistance power against disease, each person needs to maintain a lifestyle according to their body constitution and their present health condition. If a person leads a lifestyle contradictory to their natural qualities, it will diminish the vital energies (ojas, thejas, and prana) in the subtle body. For instance, if a person dominated by the earth and water elements leads a lifestyle where they sleep too long in the mornings and during the day, eat starchy and oily foods, are in a toxic relationship but are not able to leave because of attachment or depression, live in a damp place, and work in the wrong field of interest and continue in the same job, year after year, just to pay the bills, it can drain their energies and lead to severe health problems. And if a person dominant in the fire and water elements or the air and ether elements chooses the wrong lifestyle without considering their natural qualities and limitations, it will lead to bad health and cause diseases due to a weakened immune system. (You will learn more about the recommended lifestyle for each body type in chapters 12 and 13.)

7. Lack of Exercise

The human body gets its nourishment through the intake of the right foods and its rest through enough sleep. But even if a body gets food and rest, the circulatory system won't function at its optimal level without enough movement, as this is necessary for the immune cells of the body to be distributed at the maximum level. Lack of exercise can create blockages in the channels due to the accumulation of toxins, causing inflammation, and thus be an invitation to pathogens to invade the tissues of the body.

In our modern world, we restrict our body's natural movements by the items we use for our comfort in sitting, standing, and lying down. If we examine these body postures, we can see that they are not natural. For instance, if we look at our shoes, often they are far from compatible with the shape of our feet. Instead, our feet are forced to adjust to the soles and the shape of the shoes we wear. The same problem occurs with the chairs we sit on and the mattresses we sleep on. Therefore, it is important that we correct our posture and facilitate natural movements by practicing the correct yoga exercises to help us achieve maximum flexibility, balance, and strength. (You will learn more about recommended yoga programs for each body type in chapter 18.)

By establishing discipline in your daily exercise, you will improve not only your posture but also the nourishing capacity of your body by giving your circulatory system the chance to replace old cells by generating and maintaining new ones with the essence of your blood. Considering the blood as the river of your body, the carrier of nourishments in and toxins out, it is essential to support your circulatory system with the right exercise for your body type. Otherwise, a lack of exercise leads to poor blood circulation and thus weaker immunity in the cells.

As you advance in your studies of Ayurveda, you can see that different types of bodies need a different amount of, and different kinds of, exercise to maintain optimal health. For instance, while the bodies that are dominated by the earth and water elements need heavy exercise to maintain a better circulatory system, the bodies dominated by air and ether need light exercise. For the bodies dominated by the fire and water, Ayurveda recommends calming exercises to avoid disturbing the elements and thus the system. That means that in order to maintain good health and immunity, it is important not only to do exercises but also to choose the right exercises for your body type.

If you are busy in your daily life, make sure you get at least fifteen minutes of exercise every day to improve your body's natural powers. And when you have more time, perhaps on the weekends, try to do one or two hours of your complete exercise program to build up your strength, while on the other days you can maintain your health with shorter workouts.

THE THREE FORCES INFLUENCING YOUR HEALTH: KAPHA, PITTA, AND VATA

For a deeper understanding of the factors influencing our immunity and health, we now move further into the terminology of Ayurveda and how this ancient health science looks at our mind-body functions. In this chapter you will learn about birth, age, season, and time dominations and how to distinguish between prakruti and vikruti, birth dominant elements and presently dominant elements. These are words and phrases that often confuse beginners as well as longtime students of Ayurveda. You already recognize the words kapha, pitta, and vata from earlier in the book. As you read further, you will get a deeper understanding of these three forces and how people dominated by the different forces act and react in various situations in life.

· · · · · · · · · · · ·

From birth until death, a human life passes through different ages and seasons. While these changes happen in our outside nature as seasons, our inside nature, the organs and systems in our body, also change as a part of aging due to the influence of three natural forces.

Keep in mind that we all are born with five elements, but a couple of elements dominate our mind-body system from birth (conception). And during the years of our growth, external forces influence the function of our internal system, sometimes making major shifts in our dominating elements. If we don't recognize these changes in time, and make adjustments in our lifestyle accordingly, our elements can get out of balance and manifest as symptoms in the body and mind. And if we don't rectify the disturbed elements in time, they can weaken our natural resistance power and make our body prone to disease.

The very first step in maintaining your natural health and immunity is to determine your present health status using the tools of Ayurveda, and if there is an imbalance in any of the five elements, then work on balancing them. In chapter 5 you will find a self-test that will help you determine your presently dominating elements. Using those results, you can then follow the food and lifestyle recommendations given in this book for your current health condition.

Natural Factors That Affect Your Health Through Time, Age, and Seasons

Before you take the test in chapter 5 to determine your presently dominating elements (your PDE), I want to give you an idea of the factors that influence your PDE at birth and at different stages of your life. There are four factors that naturally affect our body and control our health. The very first one is the birth dominating elements that determine the core characteristics of a person's inner nature (physical and mental qualities). The birth dominating elements are the elements that dominate in a human body at the time of conception of that life in the mother's womb. Apart from the birth dominating elements, there are three more dominating factors from our outside nature that influence our immune power and health from time to time: age dominating force, season dominating force, and time of day dominating force.

The mind-body functions of a human being are influenced by the following forces:

1. The birth dominating force, which remains unchanged from birth throughout the entire life.
2. The age dominating force, which influences a person during the process of aging.
3. The season dominating force, which changes with the different seasons of the year.
4. The time dominating force, which varies during the day, from early morning until late at night.

We can look at the birth, age, season, and time clock to understand the influence of these four forces on a person's life (see illustration).

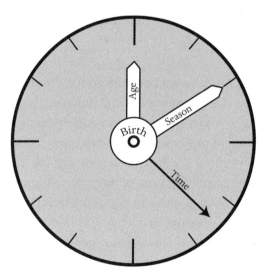

The Birth, Age, Season, and Time Clock

Natural Factors That Affect the Forces
Controlling Your Body-Mind Systems

Dominating Factor	Movement	Change in Characteristics	Shift of the Forces *(Kapha, Pitta, Pitta-Vata, and Vata, Respectively)*
Birth	No movement (permanent)	No changes during the entire life	Constant from birth until death
Age	Clockwise	Changes every thirty years	Childhood, youth, middle age, and old age
Seasons	Clockwise	Changes every three months	Spring, summer, autumn, and winter
Time of Day	Clockwise	Changes every six hours	Morning, noon, evening, and night

Our skin is the mediator between our inner and our outer nature, and if we observe the changes in our body at different ages and during different seasons of our life, we can understand the undeniable influence of Mother Nature on our health. While our inner nature (our physical organs) ages throughout the four periods of our life cycle (childhood, youth, middle age, and old age), our outer nature passes through the four seasons every year (spring, summer, fall, and winter) and influences the health of our internal systems. Besides that, the various times of day and night also influence our internal systems according to the dominating forces of those hours (morning, noon, evening, and night).

In the chart here, we can see that our birth and age dominating elements shape our characteristics from the inside, while the season and time dominating elements influence our health from the outside according to the changes in nature. That helps us understand why Ayurveda emphasizes the correlation between our health and the environment we live in.

Among these four factors, the birth dominating elements (which shape the core nature of your body) are the ones that you can change the least, and their features stay in your system throughout your life. These are the elements that have the most visible effect on your basic characteristics. (Keep in mind that no one combination of elements is better than the others. That means that whether you were born with the dominating elements of earth and water, fire and water, or air and ether, you can take advantage of your birth dominating elements and work with their unique qualities to create wellness and success in all areas of your life.)

Even though all of the elemental combinations have special qualities in a balanced state, if you forget to take care of your birth dominating elements with the right lifestyle and food for your physical body and the right mind food (thoughts) and exercise for your mental body, then while you are passing through different seasons of life, your dominating elements can become imbalanced and lead to primary symptoms such as low immunity and, in the long run, diseases in the mind-body system.

While a balanced state of the birth dominating elements supports good health and success in life, an imbalance of the elements causes physical and mental issues that need to be identified and addressed in time and corrected before they get worse. Although the greatest risk is to experience an imbalance in your birth dominating elements, sometimes you can get an imbalance in the other elements too. If you find a disturbance in any of the elements, Ayurveda recommends that you correct that imbalance before you work on the qualities of your core nature, shaped by your birth dominating elements. As an analogy, if you find a hole in a pot into which you are pouring water, first mend the hole and then fill the pot with water, as only then can you realize the maximum capacity of that pot.

Your Core Nature—The Constitutional Elements of Your Body and Mind

In the terminology of Ayurveda, our core nature is our *prakruti*, with which we are born. The word *prakruti* denotes the nature or the original state of creation. In Sanskrit, *pra* means "original" and *kruti* means "creation."

Five elements (earth, water, fire, air, and ether) create our mind-body system from the time of conception, and the three forces (kapha, pitta, and vata) formed by these fundamental elements control our physical and mental functions throughout our entire life. (We will learn more about elements and forces later in this chapter).

If you examine your mind-body system while you are healthy, you may find that some elements influence you more than others throughout your life. That is your core nature, determining your physical and mental constitution and thus your basic characteristics from the very beginning until the end of your life.

At the time of the creation of the first cell of your life in your mother's womb, the percentage of each element on the micro level of your body determines your constitutional characteristics, which is like DNA, your genetic code. During your lifetime, these dominating elements control your basic characteristics through their corresponding forces. For instance, if the percentage of the earth and water elements was higher than the percentage of the other elements at the time of conception, then the mind-body systems would be designed under the strong influence of those elements, and during their lifetime that person's physical and mental characteristics would be controlled by the force of kapha (the force that is formed by the earth and water elements). The same theory applies if the other elements have a strong influence at the time of conception, like fire and water (base of the pitta force) or air and ether (base of the vata force). This explains why the same parents can have children with different physical constitutions and mental characteristics. And this is why Ayurveda says every person is unique, even from the time of birth.

In short, we can remember the theory like this: our core characteristics, both our physical and our mental qualities, are influenced by the basic qualities of the elements that have dominated our mind-body system since birth. And our actions, both internal and external, are controlled by the dominating forces (kapha, pitta, or vata) formed by these fundamental elements that have had the greatest influence since our life began.

When you examine people with the same domination of elements, you can see that they are different in their characteristics, because the ratio of the elements differs from person to person. For example, if you study ten people with the core nature of pitta (fire and water elements), even though there are similarities in their features, you can also see that all of them are different according to the ratio of the dominating elements in their system. Or if you are considering people who have kapha (earth and water elements) or vata (air and ether elements) as their core nature, you can still see that all of them are different, even though they have some general similarities in their physical constitution and mental characteristics. If this makes sense to you, then you can understand why everybody is unique in the world.

When you are healthy, you can find your birth dominating elements by observing your deeply rooted qualities. That means that if you don't have any signals, symptoms, or diseases in your body and mind, you can identify your birth dominating elements and their actions through the dominating force in your system, which is your core, or basic, nature. In this state of balance, your birth dominating elements form the primary force of your life and apply their unique characteristics to your body and mind.

In chapter 5 you can take a self-test to find your core nature (your birth dominating elements). But prior to that, I recommend that you take the other self-test in chapter 5, the "Find Your Imbalance" test, which will tell you if any of your elements are out of balance at the moment. (As you read the following pages, you will learn why you need to determine whether you have an imbalance in any of the elements prior to finding your birth dominating elements.)

Understanding the Three Forces
in Your Inner and Outer Nature

As we have learned, the five constitutional elements in our body can only function as the three forces, which in Ayurveda terminology are known as *kapha* (earth and water elements), *pitta* (fire and water elements), and *vata* (air and ether elements). A person's core personality is shaped by the power of the dominating force in their mind-body system.

Let's take a look at these three basic forces—kapha, pitta, and vata—which determine the qualities in a human body and mind with their dominating power.

Understanding the Nature of Kapha

About two-thirds of planet Earth is water, and together with the element of earth, water forms the characteristics of kapha. To get a clear picture of the nature of kapha, think about our planet Earth, which is steady and slow in its movements, keeping everything connected with the help of gravity and following the same pattern over millions of years.

Keep these features of planet Earth in mind as you think of a person you know who has similar qualities: slow and steady in their movements; takes their time making decisions in life; feels empathy, love, and attachment to people and their surroundings; keeps the same job and follows the same lifestyle for a long period of time. If someone with similar features popped into your mind, they are a typical example of the kapha nature.

Now we can look at the basic characteristics of this core nature. A person with the kapha nature has a large bone structure and heavy muscles and a tendency to gain weight. The skin is moist, with a yellowish tone, and has an oily texture. They normally have bushy, dense hair in a darker color. The shape of the head is round and big compared to the other two natures (pitta and vata). A person with the kapha nature has large features, such as a broad forehead, a big nose, full lips, and strong and large teeth. In good health, their eyes (sclera) are clear and white. Their large, moist eyes, with bushy eyelashes and eyebrows, make them attractive and loving.

A steady appetite is one quality of this nature. The kapha nature has a pleasant body odor and strong immune power in most seasons. Normally the urine has a whitish tone, and the feces are heavy and solid.

Generally, people with the kapha nature are slow in their actions. They have a slow-grasping capacity for information coming to their mind from the outside. Although kapha dominants have a powerful memory about prior events, they often forget present matters. Their voice is heavy and they are generally slow speakers, but if you want a good listener, kapha dominants are the best choice among your friends. People dominated by the kapha force seem to have a constant and steady sex drive throughout their life.

In the area of finances, kapha dominants are savers and they guard their inherited property. People with the kapha nature seem to be successful in the caretaking fields since they like to protect everything around them. They love cooking, gardening, decorating, and being in nature. They maintain strong relationships over long periods of time and like to have deep conversations and meet with close friends. If these qualities in their constitution are out of balance, they can be too sentimental and overly attached to people and their surroundings.

People with the kapha nature can sleep deeply, and they have a hard time waking up. They experience long melancholic dreams about love or the departure of people they are close to. They are sensitive to damp climates and tend to have respiratory-related issues in those weather conditions. In a state of excess kapha, they have difficulty controlling their attachments to people and material things, and can end up with depression and eating disorders that cause obesity and related health issues.

Compared to the other two natures, kapha dominants need higher dosages of medicine for it to have an effect on their system. The pulse of a kapha dominant pulsates with the slow and steady movement of a swan.

Understanding the Nature of Pitta

We can't even imagine life without the presence of the sun. In the absence of light and warmth, we search for a glimpse of the sun, and when we catch the sunlight, we embrace that moment completely. But on the other hand, although we all love the sun, when it gets too close to us, we run away to hide from its heat. The sun is intense and hot in its basic properties. It holds the power to control the lives on our planet.

Keeping the features of the sun in mind, think about a person you know who is intense in what they do in life; is intellectual and bright like sunlight; is sharp and straight like sunrays; is brave and risk-taking; leads more than follows; and has a commanding power in speech and actions. These are some key characteristics of the force of pitta.

People with a pitta prakruti have medium bone structure and tight muscles, with a moderate weight that stays consistent, with little fluctuation. They have warm and moist skin with a pinkish-red tone. Their hair is fine and soft in texture, and they may have a tendency to go gray early or bald. They have a medium-size head with folds on the forehead, and they have penetrating eyes and fine eyelashes, a medium nose, soft red lips, pink gums, and aligned teeth. Compared to the other two natures, pitta has the strongest appetite. Their urine has a yellow color and the body odor is strong. They have a tendency to get diarrhea.

People with the pitta nature are passionate and dominating characters in their sex life. In most situations they act purposefully and with motivation. Being intellectual and demanding, they have a sharp and good memory, which helps them to be successful in their profession. They are proficient speakers, with a confident voice, and are precise in what they say. Pitta dominants tend to be successful in scientific and business fields and are interested in international affairs, news, politics, adventure and action sports, academic studies, organizing and leading groups, planning, and starting new projects and developing them into big goals. In financial matters, they spend money purposefully.

Pitta dominants generally sleep well. They fall asleep swiftly, and although they may have a tendency to wake up a few times during the night, they go right back to sleep again. Their dreams are often aggressive and about quarreling or conquering.

Since the pitta nature has hot properties, they are sensitive to sun and heat. They are prone to infection, and in a state of excess pitta, they can get skin diseases such as psoriasis, eczema, and dandruff, as well as migraines, high fever, PMS, and stomach-related issues. On the mind level, when pitta is high, they suffer from high stress and anger and get into arguments easily. If they have an enemy, they hold onto the hate with a vengeful attitude and act to destroy their opponent. Compared to the other two natures, pitta dominants require a normal dosage of medicines to heal their symptoms/diseases. The pitta nature has a frog-like, jumping pulse that helps the Vaidya determine the level of pitta in the mind-body system.

Understanding the Nature of Vata

The moon has long been a favorite of artists because of its mysterious characteristics. The moon controls the high and low tides and has qual-ities that are almost the opposite of those of the earth, such as a low level of gravity and lighter weight when compared to the earth.

See if you can think of person you know who has features similar to those of the moon: an artistic person, with a light or below-average body weight, who likes to follow their own feelings rather than the rules, enjoys travel, is always moving and making changes, and seeks freedom and loves diversity in all areas of life. These are the basic char-acteristics of the vata nature.

The body structure of a person with the vata nature differs from that of the other two (kapha and pitta). They can be tall or short, but stay slim, with a sleek bone structure, lean muscles, and thin wrists and ankles. They have difficulty gaining body weight and have a tendency to lose weight.

Compared to the other two natures, the vata domination shows up as coldness in the body tissues, such as cold hands and feet. The skin has a bluish-brown tone, and in cold climates it can get dry and rough. Blue veins can be visible under the skin on the hands and legs. They have fine hair and fragile nails. The structure of the face can be small, with features such as firm eyelashes, uneven and charming teeth, and a sleek nose, lips, and chin. Their forehead has fine lines, and their eyeballs are often unsteady, as if they are having a hard time focusing on one thing. The appetite of a vata dominant can vary in the different seasons and ages of their life. They don't sweat very much and have hardly any body odor. Their urine is plain like water, and their feces are small, with a tendency to get dry, hard, and constipated.

People with the vata nature have a habit of spending money without too much thought, and they almost always have less control over their finances than do the other two dominations. They like social gatherings and parties, traveling, meeting new people, fun games, plays, music, dance, and anything quick and brief. Most artists and creative workers are born with qualities of the vata nature.

Since the primary element of vata is air, this nature often moves fast and irregularly. The people with this nature are big dreamers, and in their sex life they hold strong desire in the mind but low energy in reality. They are fast-moving on the surface level of the mind, which shows in their instant thinking and feeling. Therefore, they remember most things in the present but easily forget the past. Since their thoughts and feelings fluctuate, they have a hard time focusing on one thing at a time. They talk about several different matters at the same time and sometimes even forget what they were just about to say.

The sleep pattern of this nature is light and interrupted. Since the moon has a direct influence on a vata-dominated body and mind, they have difficulty getting to sleep during full moon periods. They often wake up during the night and have dreams such as falling from heights or flying in the sky.

People with the vata nature are sensitive to cold and wind and have a low level of immune power in their system compared to the other two dominations. In a state of excess vata, they can have pain in the joints and mental disorders such as anxiety attacks, hysteria, fear, and shivering. They often suffer from reproductive and nervous system diseases. Ayurveda suggests the minimum dosage of medicines, since they have a rapid effect on the mind-body system of the vata nature. People with the vata nature have a pulse that resembles a slithering snake.

········· **Chapter 4** ·········

SIGNS OF BALANCE AND IMBALANCE IN THE MIND-BODY SYSTEM

When you are healthy, your symptoms disappear, your immune system functions optimally, and you feel healthy on all levels. But more than that, when you are healthy, you will also notice that your personal uniqueness, your qualities and strengths, show more than ever. In this chapter you will get an idea of which personal qualities correspond to the three forces of kapha, pitta, and vata. You will also learn what happens when the forces get high in the system and common reasons why they become aggravated.

· · · · · · · · · · · ·

Signs of Balance

As we have learned, every person is born with a greater influence of a set of elements that forms the dominating force and designs the basic characteristics of that person. In a state of balance, the qualities of your birth dominating elements, the basic features of your core nature, remain as the keys of your wellness. These key features help you understand your uniqueness, and if you know how to drive those qualities in your professional and personal lives, you can move on with ever-growing success in all areas of your life. Now let's take a look at the basic qualities of each force and their effect on your life when their corresponding elements are in a state of balance.

Kapha Qualities in Balance

Body: Strong tissues, deep breathing, moist skin, clear white eyes, good stamina

Mind: Deep spiritual interest, calm and peaceful attitude, patient, close connection to nature, loving and caring, forgiving, listening, respectful, high moral values

Pitta Qualities in Balance

Body: Good digestion and energy, clear eyes, soft skin and nails, high vitality, relaxed muscles

Mind: Enthusiastic, intelligent, independent, good leadership, friendly, courageous, pleasant, adventurous, methodical

Vata Qualities in Balance

Body: Flexible, pain-free joints, good metabolism, shiny skin and nails, balance between the left and right sides of the body, energetic, uninterrupted sleep

Mind: Creative, artistic, awake, energetic, flexible, cheerful, positive, focused, self-encouraging

Signs of Imbalance

The imbalanced state of any element can aggravate the corresponding force and interrupt the normal function of our organs, creating dysfunction in our system that, according to Ayurveda terminology, is known as *vikruti*. The state of vikruti occurs in a body when the prakruti (core nature) is disturbed. While the word *prakruti* denotes "original creation," *vikruti* stands for "after creation." The Sanskrit word *vi* means "after" and *kruti* means "creation."

As you have learned, your birth dominant elements are like your DNA: they won't change during your entire life. But with the influence of factors such as age, seasons, different times of the day and night, and other factors, your mind-body functions can fluctuate slightly from their primary characteristics, which is quite natural. However, if your primary or other forces are aggravated to more than a certain level, this can interrupt the natural functions of your mind-body system. This aggravated state is called your *vikruti*. (You can have vikruti in one, two, or even all three forces at the same time.)

If you are suffering from any symptoms or diseases or getting any signals of dysfunction from your mind-body system, it is a sign that either your birth dominating elements or any of the other elements are in a state of imbalance, and are aggravating the corresponding force or forces and causing an uneasy (dis-ease) function of an organ or even a whole system of your body or mind, or both.

Other factors influencing your body and mind, apart from birth, age, seasons, and time, are food and lifestyle. Imagine if you tried to plant a coconut tree in an arctic climate. What would happen? Even if you planted the coconut tree in a greenhouse, it wouldn't grow as it naturally does in a tropical climate. If you are following a lifestyle or food structure that is not suitable for your birth dominating elements, you will struggle to maintain your life in the wrong environment, just like the coconut tree in the greenhouse in an arctic land. Because of the wrong choices of lifestyle or food habits, your primary force or the other forces can get aggravated and give off signals of dysfunction or develop into symptoms or even diseases that affect the smooth function of your engine—your mind-body system.

Regardless of your core nature (your birth dominant elements), if you have an imbalance in any of the five fundamental elements, that will aggravate the corresponding force (or forces) and take over control of your mind-body system, creating uneasy functions of the organs. In a state of imbalance in any of the elements, the qualities of your core nature can't perform to their potential; instead, your natural skills are stifled.

Let us take a look at the common signs of imbalance in the elements and their influence on different forces, which manifest as signals, symptoms, or diseases in our mind-body system.

Prakruti vs. Vikruti

Reminder: your *prakruti* (core nature) is the result of the dominating elements at the time of your conception, which control the functions of your body and mind according to the ratio of the forces (kapha:pitta:vata). Your *vikruti* results from a disturbance in a force (or two or three forces) caused by an imbalance in one or more elements. Keep in mind that you are not your vikruti; instead, see your vikruti as a disorder of your system that can be corrected with the right food and lifestyle choices.

Signs of Earth-Water (Kapha) Imbalance

In the early stages of kapha vikruti, caused by the negligence of an imbalance in the water and earth elements in the system, the body sweats more profusely and the tone of the skin and sclera becomes yellowish and dull. Signs of excess kapha also manifest as infections and diseases in the upper part of the body, such as sinusitis and throat congestion, breathing problems, and obesity.

Extra tiredness, especially in the mornings, is a sign of too much kapha in the body. In this state, the person talks at an extremely slow pace, with a heavy voice, and takes a long time to act or react. Tonsillitis and a feeling of heaviness in the body and mind are early signs that an increased level of the kapha force is ruling the system. In this stage the person can be lazy, melancholic, sentimental, and depressed or have a desire to lead a materialistic life. Kapha vikruti also manifests in a person's behavior, such as greediness, a craving for sweets, and being overly attached to people and things.

If the heightened level of kapha is not identified and rectified in time, it can cause severe issues on the mental and physical levels. In that state, the force of kapha gets even more aggravated and drains the energy. The person can feel tired even after a long sleep. In the long run, an aggravation of the kapha force can lead to heart disease, high cholesterol and blood pressure, type 2 diabetes, and a slow-functioning immune system that can cause asthma, allergies, and other respiratory-related infections and diseases. Kapha vikruti can lead the mind to depressive thoughts and self-hatred, a complete loss of control over food and drink, and addiction to unhealthy habits and immoral activities.

Signs of Fire-Water (Pitta) Imbalance

The very first sign of pitta vikruti, caused by an imbalance in the fire and water elements in the system, is a weak immune system that allows colds and infections to enter the body. The symptoms of aggravated pitta normally begin in the middle part of the body where the digestive system functions, including the stomach, pancreas, liver, spleen, and small intestines. Hyperacidity in the stomach, a burning sensation in the esophagus and eyes, skin-related issues such as dandruff, eczema, or psoriasis, and headaches are other initial signs of an irritated pitta force.

Since the cradle of pitta is the digestive organs, any disturbance in this force causes disorders in the digestive system. Shallow breathing (a feeling of not getting enough air in the lungs) or inflammatory pain in the lumbar region can also be the beginning stage of pitta vikruti. Other signs include low blood pressure, constipation or diarrhea, irritation in the eyes, and redness in the sclera.

Heightened pitta can disturb the smooth function of the mind and lead to overambition, irritation, dissatisfaction, anger, and stress. A person with pitta vikruti often shows signs of restlessness, impatience, or unhappiness and can be demanding, dominating, manipulative, egoistic, controlling, critical, or aggressive. People in a state of excess pitta often work extra hard to make everything perfect, but are never satisfied with the final results.

After a longer period of time, these uneasy feelings can create jealousy or hatred and lead to a destructive attitude. If pitta vikruti lingers in the body, there is a risk of getting ulcers, migraines, tinnitus, eye power variations, arthritis, and thyroid gland enlargement, and in the long run it can lead to cancer in the stomach, liver, and pancreas.

Signs of Air-Ether (Vata) Imbalance

Vata vikruti, caused by an imbalance of the air and ether elements in the system, normally manifests in the lower part of the body where the reproductive organs and excretion channels are located. An excess of vata can be observed in the reactions of the body to the aggravated force, such as cold hands and feet and extra dryness in the sclera, nails, skin, and hair. Urinary infections and low back pain are also some early signs of vata vikruti. During these periods, sleep can become light or interrupted and affected by fearful dreams. The person in this state might experience disturbed focus, poor memory, a lack of confidence, and a feeling of extra tiredness. If the aggravated vata force rules the mind, the person may become anxious, superficial, unreliable, disturbed, judgmental, self-critical, or agitated and talk out of control.

In situations where the vata vikruti is neglected for a long time, the irritated force can press the mind into a state of deep anxiety, hopelessness, or feeling lost on the life path. In this stage the person might have a self-pitying and self-punishing attitude and a lack of trust. This disturbed state of vata can lead to sleep deprivation and mental difficulties such as constant fear and nervousness. These personality traits can show up in the person's speech and actions while interacting with other people. If untreated for a long period of time, excess vata can lead to issues in the reproductive organs such as the ovaries/prostate, menstrual disorders, miscarriages, or nervous disorders and severe pain in the sacral region.

Causes of Imbalance

When you go for an Ayurveda consultation, the practitioner will ask questions about your daily routines and lifestyle, including your food habits, to find out what has caused the imbalances in your system. This way the practitioner can help you not only heal your present health problems but also reduce your chances of ever facing the issues again in your life. Though several factors such as age, season, or even the time of the day can aggravate the natural forces in our mind-body system, there are other reasons we can point to as well. Let us discuss the most common factors in our daily life that can create imbalances in our elements and aggravate the forces, weakening our immune system and decreasing life energy.

> Although there is a greater chance that our birth dominating elements will become out of balance, the other elements can also become imbalanced because of the choices we make when it comes to food and lifestyle.

Causes of Kapha Aggravation

We know that the kapha force is slow in action, steady in its position, and restricted in its movements. Without understanding these basic characteristics, if a person with this core nature leads a life in slow motion, following the course of this force, it will increase the kapha and the person will become more and more slow as the years go by.

Since kapha is highly influencing in the morning, if a person with a kapha core nature has a habit of waking up late, this can heighten the force of kapha even further. For a person with this core nature, even a nap during the day can lead to heaviness and dullness in the body and mind. If this person is not moving physically and is not active mentally during the day, the systems can show signs of an earth and water imbalance and aggravate the corresponding force of kapha.

People with the kapha nature have an attachment tendency, so accumulating material things and following unhealthy routines will increase the force of kapha and eventually make these people slaves to these habits.

As we will learn later in this book, any kind of food that is sweet, sour, or salty in its basic qualities can increase the force of kapha. Certain habits can also increase kapha, including eating too late in the evening and too early in the morning, treating food as a companion when the mind is disturbed by sentimental or depressed feelings, and overeating. Foods that are heavy, cold, and oily create an imbalance in the earth and water elements, especially for people with this core nature. All kinds of chilled drinks, ice cream, and fried foods such as french fries also aggravate kapha.

Causes of Pitta Aggravation

With the opposite characteristics of the kapha force, pitta is fast in action, determined in its position, and prompt in its movements. If someone with pitta as their core nature tries to take advantage of these basic qualities without knowing the "brakes" or limits of pitta, this force will accelerate to the highest and finally run into a wall, causing an imbalance in the fire and water elements that aggravates the force of pitta in the mind-body system.

Since people with the pitta force as their core nature are sensitive to heat, too much exposure to sharp and direct sunlight or being in conditions with excessive heat can cause related health issues. People with the pitta core nature can have a tendency to be workaholics, and when they are engaged in something, they may forget to take enough breaks and not eat on time, which irritates the force of pitta.

Since pitta has hot properties, eating sour, pungent, or salty foods can increase the fire in the digestive system and aggravate this force. Other habits such as the use of alcohol or tobacco and eating processed sweets or deep-fried or very spicy foods can also increase the level of pitta. Since pitta is on time and functions like a clock, skipping a meal or eating at irregular times can affect the digestive system and cause health issues in the long run.

Drinking less during the day and eating while holding feelings of anger, irritation, or disappointment are also major reasons for excess pitta. Since the force of pitta maintains good health by supporting the immune system with the help of agni and jalam, the fire and water elements, any imbalance in these elements will directly disturb the force of pitta and weaken the immune power, leading to symptoms such as lower blood values, fatigue syndrome, autoimmune disorders, and stomach dysfunction.

Causes of Vata Aggravation

The vata force is quick in action, indecisive in its position, and continuous but unsteady in its movements. In the absence of this knowledge, if someone lives with vata as their core nature and moves forward following the natural course of vata, this force can generate a tempest instead of a breeze in the mind-body system, causing an imbalance in the air and ether elements that heightens the force of vata and its related symptoms.

People with vata as their core nature are generally sensitive to cold and turbulent situations. The vata force has a high chance of getting aggravated if these people do not take care of their body with warm food and appropriate clothing in the cold season, do not get enough rest and relaxation by overworking, do not go to bed on time, or engage in nightlife or late-night activities. Also, being in loud and noisy environments and using alcohol and tobacco can create an imbalance in the air and ether elements. Strenuous and frantic activities such as hard exercise and extremely adventurous sports can also disturb this force.

Since vata is cold, dry, and light in its basic properties, eating ice cream, chips, or popcorn, especially during a highly vata-influencing time like in the evening, increases the movement of this force. And even though bitter food has medicinal value, it can heighten the force of vata if overused. Food that tastes astringent and pungent is also vata-stimulating. All frozen or cold foods and drinks can lead to issues in the lower digestive system, such as the colon, which is controlled primarily by the force of vata.

Even healthy food can cause gastric trouble in the lower abdominal area of vata dominants if it is prepared without spices that support digestion. That is why uncooked food seems to be a little harder to digest for a person with vata as their core nature, even though raw food is one of the best sources of nourishment. But from my experience, if vata dominants carefully choose the right ingredients and eat foods with the right spices and in a warm atmosphere, even raw plant-based food can work without creating stomach issues.

Certain habits, such as eating irregularly or skipping meals, eating smaller quantities of food than what the body needs, and eating or drinking while holding a feeling of fear or anxiousness, can also disturb the force of vata and cause related health issues. When vata is high, it weakens the immune system and manifests in the form of cold feet and palms, dry, itchy skin, and inflammation in the body, especially in the joints and pelvic region.

How to Balance an Imbalance

If you find a vikruti in your mind-body system, you can correct the aggravated force with the help of the right food and lifestyle disciplines. Before starting your disciplines, you need to know the following:

1. To start your Ayurveda practice, first find your PDE: the presently dominating elements that form the leading force in your system and control your mind-body system. You can find your PDE by taking the self-tests in chapter 5.

2. The first self-test in chapter 5, "Find Your Imbalance," will tell you whether you have a vikruti (imbalance) in your system. If you don't have an imbalance in your system at present, you will get zero points on this test. In other words, if you don't have any signals, symptoms, or diseases in your body and mind at the moment, it means that your fundamental elements are in a state of equilibrium and are not disturbing any of the three forces in your mind-body system. In this case, you can move on to the next self-test, "Find Your Core Nature," to find your prakruti (your birth dominating elements) and follow the recommendations accordingly to maintain the balance in your system. But if you answer yes to any of the questions in the first test, then your PDE (your presently dominating elements) is considered to be your vikruti, which means that you have an imbalance in the dominating elements that is aggravating the corresponding force (or forces) in your mind-body system, causing your present symptoms/diseases, which need to be taken into consideration primarily.

3. If you do the "Find Your Imbalance" test in chapter 5 and find that your PDE is your *prakruti*, then you can maintain the balance of your birth dominating elements with the Ayurveda disciplines in this book to maintain your perfect health. But if you find that your PDE is your *vikruti*, then it is

possible that your PDE and your prakruti differ, which might make you confused about which Ayurveda recommendations to follow and what to balance first—your prakruti or your vikruti. Keep in mind that you should always follow the recommendations to balance your PDE, regardless of whether it is your prakruti or your vikruti.

In the first part of our studies, we learned about the major forces that influence our health and immunity. While your birth dominating elements and their corresponding force are constant throughout your life, the dominating forces of age, seasons, and time of day change and influence your health over time. We also learned the basic characteristics of each force (kapha, pitta, and vata) and their effect on our health in a stable state and an aggravated state.

Next, with the help of a self-test, you are going to find your PDE: the presently dominating elements that form the leading force in your system and control your mind-body functions. As per the test results, you can follow the lifestyle and food recommendations in the coming chapters to maintain the balance of your dominating elements and forces and thus your optimal health and immunity.

YOUR PDE (PRESENTLY DOMINATING ELEMENTS)— THE BLUEPRINT OF YOUR HEALTH

Now that you are familiar with the basic theory and terminology of Ayurveda, it is time to start using this wisdom in your daily life to boost your immune power and regain your natural health. In this chapter you will find two self-tests that will tell you where to start your practice. Make sure you read the instructions and be honest with yourself while filling out the tests, keeping in mind that the accuracy and helpfulness of the test results depends on your truthful answers.

· · · · · · · · · · · · ·

To begin your Ayurveda practice, first you need to find your PDE, the presently dominating elements in your mind-body system, which is like the blueprint of your current state of health. Your PDE represents either your core nature (shaped by your birth dominating elements) or your imbalanced elements (aggravating the corresponding force, and causing your major health issues at present). The highest dominating force in your mind-body system at the moment is your PDE, regardless of whether it is your prakruti (birth dominating elements) or your vikruti (presently dominating elements).

Self-Tests to Determine Your Present Health Status

Remember that if any of the five elements is out of balance and is disturbing your mind-body system through the associated force in the form of a signal, symptom, or disease, that is the area you need to work on first to get back into balance. With the help of the "Find Your Imbalance" test, let us find out whether or not you have an imbalance in your system at the moment.

The force that gets the most points in the "Find Your Imbalance" test is the force that is currently most aggravated in your system, and this is what you need to focus on right now, to balance the corresponding elements with the right Ayurveda food and lifestyle disciplines. (Remember that one or two or sometimes all three forces can be aggravated, which manifests as different symptoms and issues. However, we need to start with the most urgent health issues and address the other issues later, step-by-step. That is why you always need to follow the recommendations for your most severely disturbed force, which you can identify at the end of the test by the total number points you tally for each force.)

When you follow the Ayurveda recommendations in this book according to the test results, you can notice gradual changes in your health after about three weeks. If you adapt the food and lifestyle changes according to your PDE and practice in a disciplined way, then you can retake the test every three months until your imbalances are under control.

When your answer for all the questions in the "Find Your Imbalance" test is no, it means that your body and mind are in good health and you are at the top of your natural resistance power. Then you can move on to the "Find Your Core Nature" test to understand your birth dominant elements and follow the Ayurveda recommendations to support the stability of your core nature. This will help you maintain your present health and resistance power and help prevent you from getting sick in the future as well. If you answer all the questions accurately in the "Find Your Core Nature" test, then the force that gets the most points will be the force that was dominant over the other two forces at the time of your birth and that built the base of the primary qualities in your body and mind.

How to Do the "Find Your Imbalance" Test

- Read and contemplate each question and circle Y (Yes) or N (No) at the end of the sentence.

- Simply select whether your mind says yes or no to a question, without judging or criticizing yourself.

- Finally, calculate the total number of points for each force by comparing the questions you selected "Y" for with the key in the section at the end of the book called "Tallying Your Test Results."

- The force with the highest number of points is your primary imbalance: the presently dominating elements in your system. Start working on reducing your most aggravated force by balancing your PDE with the lifestyle recommendations in this book.

- Take the "Find Your Imbalance" test again after three months, and follow the recommendations according to the result.

- Continue to do the "Find Your Imbalance" test every three months until you get zero points for all three forces. Then move on to the "Find Your Core Nature" test.

- Keep in mind that regardless of your age and your present health condition, your aim is to have *zero* issues in your system in the future. To make it practical, break down this goal into three-month periods, and with the practice of Ayurveda for your presently dominating elements, move forward until you achieve your perfect health. Once you achieve your perfect health, then maintain it with the Ayurveda disciplines for your PDE.

TEST 1: Find Your Imbalance

During the past three weeks, have you:

1. experienced unusually cold hands and feet, even indoors? Y / N
2. experienced excess body heat that is not caused by climatic conditions or physical activity? Y / N
3. experienced extra dry skin, nails, and hair? Y / N

4. experienced skin diseases such as dandruff or eczema? Y/N

5. had yellowish eyes and skin? Y/N

6. experienced a burning sensation in your eyes and skin? Y/N

7. had psoriasis? Y/N

8. experienced alopecia? Y/N

9. experienced excessive fatigue during the midday, especially after lunch? Y/N

10. experienced extra tiredness in the morning for more than two successive days? Y/N

11. felt tired even after a long sleep? Y/N

12. been very slow in your speech, actions, and reactions? Y/N

13. experienced poor short-term memory? Y/N

14. had recurring headaches? Y/N

15. experienced migraines or tinnitus? Y/N

16. experienced a rapid decline in eye power? Y/N

17. experienced excessive gas in the bowels? Y/N

18. experienced constipation? Y/N

19. experienced high acid levels in the stomach, including acid reflux or heartburn? Y/N

20. experienced joint pain? Y/N

21. experienced inflammation or pain in the thoracic or lumbar region of your spine? Y/N

22. experienced back pain in the sacrum or coccyx? Y/N

23. experienced excessive sweating? Y/N

24. been overweight? Y/N

25. experienced low blood pressure? Y/N

26. had high blood pressure? Y/N

27. been diagnosed with high cholesterol levels? Y/N

28. experienced mucus congestion in the throat? Y/N

29. had sinusitis? Y/N

30. had bronchitis? Y/N

31. had asthma? Y/N

32. experienced urinary infections? Y/N

33. had osteoarthritis? Y/N

34. had rheumatoid arthritis? Y/N

35. experienced hyperthyroidism? Y/N

36. experienced hypothyroidism? Y/N

37. had a miscarriage? Y/N

38. had type 2 diabetes? Y/N

39. had a heart disease? Y/N

40. had light or interrupted sleep on a consistent basis? Y/N

41. been experiencing insomnia? Y/N

42. been feeling restless or stressed? Y/N

43. been feeling gloomy or sentimental? Y/N

44. been feeling lazy? Y/N

45. had cravings for sweets? Y/N

46. been feeling ungrounded? Y/N

47. been feeling nervous? Y/N

48. been feeling worried? Y/N

49. been feeling fearful? Y/N

50. been experiencing anxiety? Y/N

51. been experiencing low self-confidence? Y/N

52. been feeling inferior and self-judgmental? Y/N

53. been feeling judgmental toward others? Y/N

54. been experiencing self-loathing? Y/N

55. experienced difficulty in keeping promises? Y/N

56. been feeling unfocused? Y/N

57. been feeling confused and uncertain? Y/N

58. been experiencing mistrust because of low self-confidence? Y/N

59. been feeling frustrated or irritated? Y/N

60. been argumentative or accusing? Y/N

61. been domineering or controlling? Y/N

62. been demanding or manipulative? Y/N

63. been egotistical or selfish? Y/N

64. been materialistic or greedy? Y/N

65. felt overly attached to people or things? Y/N

66. been stuck in old patterns or memories? Y/N

67. been feeling melancholic? Y/N

68. been feeling burned out by stress? Y/N

69. been extremely critical? Y/N

70. had a destructive or vengeful attitude? Y/N

71. been feeling hateful or jealous? Y/N

72. experienced uncontrolled anger? Y/N

73. engaged in self-harming behavior? Y/N

74. been anorexic? Y/N

75. been feeling lethargic or lifeless? Y/N

76. been having suicidal thoughts? Y/N

77. been feeling depressed or isolating yourself? Y/N

78. been eating or drinking without being able to stop? Y/N

79. been engaging in immoral behavior? Y/N

80. been abusive? Y/N

81. engaged in any form of psychopathic behavior? Y/N

82. had a nervous disorder? Y/N

83. been hysterical? Y/N

84. engaged in any form of tyrannical behavior? Y/N

85. been obese? Y/N

86. had extreme obesity? Y/N

87. had reddish sclera? Y/N

88. During the past six months, have you been diagnosed with ovarian or prostate cancer? Y/N

89. During the past six months, have you been diagnosed with stomach or liver cancer? Y/N

90. During the past three months, have you experienced any menstrual disorders apart from premenstrual syndrome (PMS)? Y/N

91. During the past three months, have you experienced pronounced symptoms of premenstrual syndrome (PMS)? Y/N

How to Do the "Find Your Core Nature" Test

Please keep in mind that you should be free from imbalances before taking the "Find Your Core Nature" test, since an imbalance in any element can distort your answers and give a faulty picture of your birth dominating elements.

- Read and contemplate each question and all the potential answers in the "Find Your Core Nature" test before circling the option that best describes you.

- Don't skip any question. If two answers come close for the same question, choose the one that is closest to your personality.

- If it's still difficult to choose just one answer, then find the answers with the help of your best friend, who might know you better than you know yourself.

- When you're done with the test, calculate the total number of points for each force using the key in the section at the end of the book called "Tallying Your Test Results."

- The force with the highest number of points is your core nature (the dominating elements at your birth), which is also your PDE (presently dominating elements).

- Follow the lifestyle recommendations for your PDE to continue to maintain the balance of your elements and your wellness and natural immune power throughout the coming seasons and ages.

- If you experience a symptom in your mind-body system at any time in your life, you can go back and take the "Find Your

Imbalance" test again to determine which elements have disturbed your system and start work accordingly on your PDE to get back into balance.

TEST 2: Find Your Core Nature

Answer each question:

1. Which best describes your mind?

    X. Caring, loving, forgiving, calm, supportive, peaceful, slow to grasp but steady.

    Y. Intelligent, brave, stubborn, independent, focused, perfectionist, critical.

    Z. Creative, spontaneous, flexible, uplifting, curious, fast but shallow.

2. Which best describes your preferred activities?

    X. International affairs, news, politics, adventures and action sports, academic studies, organizing and leading groups, planning projects and setting goals.

    Y. Cooking, gardening, taking care of and beautifying people and things (like houses), being in water, being in nature, having deep conversations and meetings with close friends.

    Z. Social gatherings and parties, traveling, meeting new people, quick and short activities, fun games, plays, dance, and music.

3. Which best describes your mood?

    X. Shifting quickly between feeling energetic and dispirited, happy and unhappy, positive and negative.

    Y. Low energy in the morning and higher in the evening, stable, slow changes from one mood to another.

    Z. Energetic, enthusiastic, adventurous, highest energy in the morning and low in the evening.

4. Which best describes your memory?

    X. Sharp and good memory.

    Y. Poor long-term memory and good short-term memory, forgets easily.

    Z. Strong long-term memory and poor short-term memory.

5. Which best describes your talents/interests?

    X. Caretaking/preservation, production.

    Y. Business/sales, leadership.

    Z. Art/design, entertainment.

6. Which best describes your spending habits?

    X. Purposeful spender.

    Y. Big saver, with a habit of protecting inherited property.

    Z. Big spender, with less control over finances.

7. Which best describes your sleep and dreams?

    X. Deep sleep; hard to wake up; long, flowing, melancholic dreams, usually about love or being left by close people.

    Y. Moderate sleep, falls asleep immediately but tends to wake up sometimes, aggressive dreams of quarrels or conquering.

    Z. Tendency toward light, interrupted sleep; has difficulty falling asleep and often wakes up; nightmares about falling or uncertain situations.

8. Which best describes your actions?

    X. Tempo varies and changes quickly.

    Y. Motivated and purposeful.

    Z. Slow and steady, high endurance.

9. Which best describes your sex drive?

    X. Devoted and constant.

    Y. Dominating and passionate.

    Z. Strong desire but low energy.

10. Which best describes your appetite?

> X. Changeable.
>
> Y. Regular.
>
> Z. Strong.

11. Which best describes your digestion?

> X. Slow.
>
> Y. Fast.
>
> Z. Irregular.

12. Which of the following types of weather are you most sensitive to?

> X. Sun and heat.
>
> Y. Wind and cold.
>
> Z. Humid and damp.

13. Which best describes your voice and speech?

> X. Hoarse or high-pitched or quiet voice, nervous and quick speech, often forgets the key points.
>
> Y. Loud and sharp voice, confident and precise speech, gets to the point directly.
>
> Z. Soft, deep, and calm voice; deep and emotional speech; good listener and slow speaker.

14. Which best describes your skin type?

> X. Tends to be cold and moist or oily, with a hint of yellowish-white.
>
> Y. Sensitive to heat and sun, a hint of pinkish-red, warm and moist.
>
> Z. Cold and rough, a hint of bluish-brown, tends to be dry.

15. Which best describes your hair and nails?

    X. Fine and soft hair, early gray or bald; soft, oily, shiny nails with flexible cuticles.

    Y. Thin and silky hair; thin, brittle, dry nails with rough cuticles.

    Z. Dense, bushy, and dark hair; strong, thick, shiny nails with soft cuticles.

16. Which best describes your facial structure?

    X. Small head with fine lines on forehead, thin and firm eyelashes, sleek nose, thin lips, small chin, irregular teeth.

    Y. Medium-size head with folds on forehead, fine eyelashes, medium nose, soft and red lips, pink gums and regular teeth.

    Z. Big, round head with a broad forehead; large, bushy eyebrows; big nose and large, soft lips; aligned, large teeth with oily gums.

17. Which best describes your eyes?

    X. Steady, sharp eyes.

    Y. Unsteady/irregular movements of irises.

    Z. Large, moist eyes.

18. Which best describes your body structure?

    X. Asymmetrical body (top and bottom); large bone structure and heavy muscle structure.

    Y. Symmetrical body; medium bone structure and firm muscle structure.

    Z. Asymmetrical body (left and right sides); thin bone structure and slim muscle structure.

19. Which best describes your weight?

    X. Low—tendency to carry less weight.

    Y. Moderate—quite steady weight.

    Z. Heavy—tendency to be overweight.

20. Which best describes your body odor?

> X. Mild/sweet smell.
>
> Y. Strong smell.
>
> Z. Subtle/indistinct smell.

21. Which best describes your urine?

> X. Colorless.
>
> Y. Whitish.
>
> Z. Yellow

Part 2

FOOD—
YOUR NATURAL MEDICINE

Ayurveda teaches us three natural practices in our daily life to maintain optimal health and immunity in all seasons and at all ages. These basic disciplines to stabilize the functions of the mind-body system are considered the three commandments of this ancient health science, and in Sanskrit they are known as *aahar* (food), *vihar* (lifestyle) and *vijar* (thoughts).

As an old saying in my village goes, your health is your choice and your happiness is your birthright, which literally becomes true when you learn about the three commandments of Ayurveda and practice them in your daily life. When you take responsibility for these three vital areas of your life, you can lead your mind with affirmative thoughts and your lifestyle with healthy disciplines, including diet, exercise, and relaxation programs. And when you know what to feed your brain and your stomach and how to use your precious time on this planet to make the most of your present life, good fortune will follow in your footsteps, and health and happiness will reside in your body and mind as conscious choices for the rest of your life. Then the question is, if this ancient health science works perfectly in our life, why is our society not using Ayurveda as a mainstream life practice?

There are a few reasons that Ayurveda is not yet widely received in our modern world. From my experience, I can tell you that these reasons are based in misconceptions about this ancient health science. While some people believe that there is no scientific evidence behind this health wisdom, others believe this ancient practice might limit their modern lifestyle and comforts. Since our present world gauges the value of everything with the scale of science, I can understand this argument, but I must ask, what outside evidence do you need that is more important than the results from your own life practice?

As a public speaker working around the world as an ambassador of Ayurveda for the last two decades, I hear not only uplifting voices but also sometimes offensive questions and comments from the public. Once I heard a scientist say that Ayurveda is mumbo-jumbo, which simply means that, in his opinion, there is no practical value to this health science in our modern world. After listening to his argument, I responded that if you can't believe in the healing powers of Ayurveda, that is fine, but before closing the door to this life wisdom, ask yourself, isn't it better to believe in something that is mumbo-jumbo and feel good in your mind and body than to live in a state of stress and dissatisfaction your entire life?

I haven't written about anything in this book that hasn't shown results or that I haven't proven myself. From my experience in working with all kinds of people on different continents, I can tell you that Ayurveda will upgrade your life to the next level. This wisdom can help you choose the best of everything in life, whether it is your food practice, lifestyle disciplines, or mind development.

When you practice Ayurveda, you live with consciousness. So you take control by choosing everything that matches with your life and is the best for your health. By making these important choices in your life, you become the leader of your mind, instead of being a servant obeying the orders of unhealthy habits and addictions. Through the continuous practice of this health wisdom, you are not only choosing your food and your thoughts but also gaining the power to make choices in all areas of your life.

In the coming sections of this book, we will look at how we can make use of the Ayurveda disciplines by our conscious choices in life. We will begin our studies by gaining an understanding of the terms *aahar* (food) in part 2 and *vihar* (lifestyle) in part 3, and learning how these disciplines can be applied to your health routines to enhance your immunity. At the end of the book, I'll also give you an introduction to the term *vijar* (thoughts) for your mental development.

When you understand the possibilities of upgrading your health with the tools of Ayurveda, you can make conscious choices in your daily life based on your present health status. By knowing the PDE (presently dominating elements) of your mind-body system, you can redesign your diet, lifestyle, and the functions of your mind, and work on your health to attain the maximum benefit of your core nature, your constitutional qualities hidden in your personality since birth. Once you understand the qualities and limitations of your inner nature, you can then learn about the correlation between your internal systems and your outer nature. In the coming chapters, you will also learn how your body acts with and reacts to changes in nature, with the varying seasons and times of day, and how you can tune your mind-body system to function with ease (instead of dis-ease), promoting perfect health and maintaining maximum resistance power and vitality.

Since the beginning of our life on this planet, food has been treated as a natural medicine that nurtures, cleanses, and heals our body in all seasons and at all ages. Through the food we eat every day, we receive nutrients in our body as proteins, carbohydrates, minerals, vitamins, and fatty acids, which are essential for building new cells—the building blocks of our body.

A human body is a composition of trillions of cells, and the health and immune power of a person depends upon the maintenance of these micro units of life through the right nourishment. These tiny cells form our tissues, the tissues form organs, the sets of organs form systems, and finally the different systems together form our complex body.

According to Ayurveda terminology, the human body is formed with seven *dhatus*—seven sets of tissues. In Sanskrit, these seven tissues are known as *rasa* (lymph), *rakta* (blood), *mamsa* (muscle), *medha* (fat), *asthi* (bone), *majja* (bone marrow), and *shukra* (reproductive tissue). The status of these tissues determines a body's health and immunity.

With the help of *sama agni*, the balanced state of the fire element, a healthy body maintains good digestion, proper absorption of nutrients at the cellular level, and the elimination of waste particles from the system. But these three functions of the body—digestion, absorption, and elimination—depend not only on the natural functions of the internal systems but also on the food we take into our stomach every day.

If a person merely feeds their stomach without considering their present health condition or blindly follows an addiction to unhealthy food and drink, then even if they naturally have a healthy digestive system with a sama agni (balanced fire), eventually the digestion will collapse, creating stomach issues. These symptoms will manifest as acid reflux, hyperacidity, gas, bloating, or slow or difficult digestion, depending on the level of disturbed agni in the system.

Because of our poor food choices, our digestion and metabolism fail, and the agni in the system gets out of balance, weakening our immunity. Considering these facts, we can see the importance of maintaining a healthy diet to support the performance of our internal systems at an optimal level. When you avoid unhealthy food by incorporating nature's pure essence as your daily food, you are one step closer to perfect health. In the coming days, you can cultivate healthy food habits by using logic and determination. And as the next step, you can watch your body and mind through the window of Ayurveda and choose the *right* foods according to your PDE, your presently dominating elements.

When you change your diet according to your present mind-body condition, you begin to see improvements in your health, which reflect internally through the smooth, dis-ease-free function of your organs and externally through your radiant skin and bright eyes.

By learning about Ayurveda, we understand that everything that goes inside our skin influences our health and immunity, and among them our daily food plays a major role. From a holistic point of view, we receive two kinds of food from the outside: mental food and physical food.

Physical Food

As we already know, we receive our physical energy through the food that is broken down in our digestive system as proteins, carbohydrates, minerals, vitamins, and fatty acids. As a part of our metabolic function, nutrients from the digested food are absorbed through the walls of the small intestines and transported throughout the bloodstream. After undergoing the filtration process in the liver, the nutrients eventually reach the micro units of our body, our cells. With the help of these nutrients, the force of kapha generates new cells, while the force of vata makes space for this creation by destroying old cells. The role of pitta is to maintain the body cells with its fire and water elements and sustain the natural immunity of the system.

Mental Food

Consider everything that our mind consumes through its five senses as our mental food, the external source of mental energy. The status of our mental immunity depends on the metabolism of our mind—the overall function of our thoughts, feelings, and emotions generated and circulated in our mental body.

To get a clear picture of our mind metabolism, let us imagine our brain as the virtual mouth of our mind and the thoughts we process as the virtual food of our mind. While the information collected by our brain through our senses forms our thoughts, the processed thoughts are swallowed down into our virtual stomach, our heart, generating our feelings. In a later stage, some of these feelings continue down to the virtual intestines of our mind and stay there as emotions, which occasionally trigger our brain to form thoughts that may or may not have any direct connection to the information from outside, collected by our five senses.

Our mind metabolism comprises different stages, such as receiving information through the senses, forming thoughts in the brain, processing the thoughts in the heart as feelings, and storing them in the lower abdomen as emotions. If we receive positive information by filtering out the negative information, or if we practice creating positive thoughts by not encouraging negativity in our brain, or cleanse the negative feelings and emotions existing in our heart and lower abdomen, then we can maintain a healthy mind by maintaining a high level of mental resistance power against the most common mental illnesses, such as heavy anxiety, uncontrolled stress, and depression—which, if untreated, will also affect our physical health and immunity. In the meditation chapters in part 4 of this book, you can read more about the function of the mind and try some of the mind exercises I give to my clients.

Chapter 6

THREE STEPS TO A HEALTHY, HAPPY STOMACH

Starting a healthy life means nourishing new habits in our daily life and becoming conscious of everything connected to our health, among which our diet plays a major role. To maintain optimal health and immunity, we need to invest enough time in discovering the best sources of nature's healing food, from the time it is harvested in the farmer's field until it reaches our stomach. To find the best sources of food and how best to ingest it into our body, we will focus on the three major areas of our food practice: shopping, cooking, and eating.

Smart Shopping

Next time you enter a supermarket, try to remind yourself that everything in the shop is there to sell but not necessarily to buy. That means you need to choose the food items that are best for your present health condition. The question is, how do you know what is best for you when there are hundreds of products stacked on the racks in front of you? Here you need to use some logic and the knowledge you have gained through your study of Ayurveda, and consider the fact that most of the products displayed in the store in attractive packages are not for you. To find the best foods for your mind-body system, you can use the information in chapter 9, which details what is best for your presently dominating elements. And according to your PDE, you can select your food, the maintainer of your natural health, using the food chart in chapter 11. But to make sure you are buying the best foods from the best sources, you need to consider a few factors before putting the items in your shopping cart.

1. *Start with the right planning.* Plan your food and drink for the next few days or a week in advance, and keep track of your healthy and unhealthy habits. I suggest that you use a notebook to write down each week's food plan and figure out which kinds of food and drink you need to increase, cut down on, or add to provide better health for your body. And as the next step, you can adjust your shopping list according to your PDE, which will help you balance the elements and bring you to optimal health.

2. *Buy health, not addiction.* This is a very interesting factor about the health of our society. Most of the time we shop not for the products that our body needs but for the products that our mind is drawn to. This happens because of our addiction to these products. When I look at the food habits of some of my clients who constantly struggle with health issues because of what they eat and drink, I can see that many of them do not even realize they have an addiction (or several addictions) that controls their shopping list. When these clients ask me what they should eat to feel better and regain their good health, I tell them to think about what they shouldn't eat rather than what to eat—which means that most of our health problems are caused by what we eat, not by what we haven't eaten.

3. *Find the origin of your food.* The source of your food is one of the most important things to check. You get the maximum nutritional value from food items that are grown close to your area and transported to the store over a short distance

and period of time. Keep in mind that most things that have to be transported a long way from the farmer's field to your plate need some kind of preservatives to keep them fresh and attractive. This is perhaps good for the grocery store, since it makes the display look fresh, but it is not good for your stomach, because it will have to digest and distribute the chemicals to your system. If you are buying an apple or a tomato, make sure it has not traveled a long way after being picked. In short, try to support local farmers and food suppliers by giving preference to their products in your shopping. This will not only improve your health but also help the environment by reducing the pollution from the transportation of the products.

4. *Health first and good deals second.* Even though we believe that we are living in a society where the consumer decides what to purchase, this is not completely true. Most of the time our brain is manipulated by the marketing tactics of multinational companies, who are actually the ones that determine our consumption habits. They can make us want to buy a product, or more of their products, by supplying attractive offers that are hard for the typical customer to pass up. So we often end up filling our shopping cart with more than we need, and as a result we use these products more than we otherwise would. In these situations we need to use our intelligence and ask ourselves if we really need these products or if we are buying them because of the special offer rather than our actual requirements. This consideration is important, especially in our food selection, since most of the time it is the unhealthy food items that come with tempting offers for the customer to grab without thinking too much.

5. *Find your addiction in your shopping cart.* All six tastes have their own properties, and the right use of the tastes leads to good health and vitality. But if we overuse any of the six tastes in our daily food and drink habits, it can cause serious health issues eventually. For instance, sweet is one taste that

is often misused in our society because of its natural ability to make us feel love and happiness. But if we use sweets to fill our heart with love and its related feelings, eventually we will get addicted to that taste, which will make everything worse, and we might end up with fatigue, depression, or related problems such as type 2 diabetes, low immunity, or obesity. This scenario applies if we use any taste in excess, like salt, pungent, sour, or even bitter. As you will learn in chapter 8, sugar and salt increase the force of kapha, pungent and sour increase pitta, and bitter and astringent increase the force of vata.

6. *Our ignorance is the food companies' profit.* Remember that knowledge is the fundamental wealth of a human, and in the context of food, that is absolutely true. Many diseases enter our body or generate in our system through the food and drink we take in, and most times we don't realize what is included in the food that we buy from the store. Of course, if you are not a farmer eating the food from your own field, it is hard to know a hundred percent about all food items. But there are ways to gain more knowledge of what our food contains if we invest some time when we purchase a packaged food item from the store. In the United States, food additives are controlled by the FDA (Food and Drug Administration) and listed on the package by their chemical names, while in the European Union they are regulated by the EFSA (European Food Safety Authority) and listed on the package as codes called E numbers (see chart). Next time you buy a packaged food item, you can look on the back of the package to see how many E numbers are in that item.

E numbers, per the European Food Safety Authority:
E100 to E199—Coloring additives
E200 to E299—Preservatives
E300 to E399—Antioxidants, acidity regulators
E400 to E499—Thickeners, stabilizers, emulsifiers
E500 to E599—Acidity regulators, anti-caking agents
E600 to E699—Flavour enhancers
E700 to E799—Antibiotics
E900 to E999—Glazing agents, gases, and sweeteners
E1000 to E1599—Additional chemicals

Keep in mind that these additives are used in food not to boost our health but to prolong the life of the product and make it look fresh until it reaches our stomach. Though most additives are certified as safe in a certain amount, it is not yet known how safe they are to our body when it comes to combinations of chemicals, their reactions in our systems, and their side effects. Looking at the long list of these additives slowly invading our system, you can understand why I encourage you to eat directly from nature and buy from local farmers as much as possible. I realize that nowadays we live in a society where it is hard to find food directly from nature, and to some extent we have to depend on packaged food. So how can we prevent these additives from reaching our stomach? My suggestion is that you always check the label on the package and buy the foods and drinks that have no additives, or choose foods with the least amount of additives in them. If I need to buy a food item that comes in a package, I try to buy the one with the fewest E numbers, and I hardly ever buy products with more than one or two additives.

The small decisions we make in our daily life have a big impact on our health. Just like the tiny raindrops that eventually fill the oceans, even a little bit of health consciousness can lead to vast changes in your overall health.

I always prefer to invest in the search for healthy food options in every new city I visit. And apart from discovering local food items, I am also interested in studying the patterns of my fellow customers at the store. You can distinguish between three dominant personalities in a supermarket even from the moment they enter the shop and choose their shopping basket. Kapha dominants usually favor the biggest steel cart, and they amble along the aisles, studying everything as they go. Pitta dominants enter the shop in a hurry, grab the smallest shopping basket, and rush toward the racks as if they already know exactly what they want to buy. The third personality type, the vata dominants, usually take a while to decide what to buy, and they usually end up choosing a medium-size plastic basket on wheels, which they pull behind them, picking items randomly.

You can see that we all have some set patterns, even in our shopping habits, so next time you are doing your grocery shopping, observe your own patterns in choosing your food, and make sure you are not buying too much or too little, but just enough items and those that are right for your PDE, your presently dominating elements.

Healthy Cooking

Cooking is a healing art, and if we understand the logic behind which type of food preparation suits our current health condition, we can say that our pharmacology starts in our kitchen. From now on, consider your kitchen as the storeroom of your own natural medicines, and see yourself as the pharmacologist of your own health issues as well as those of your whole family. With this picture in mind, how should you prepare each meal: your breakfast, lunch, dinner, and the snacks in between?

First of all, consider your present health condition. If you are suffering from any kind of illness or receiving signals from your body indicating symptoms of a dysfunctional organ or even an entire system, that is what you need to take into account when designing your diet. Simply following a trendy diet, even if it is healthy, won't help you rectify the root cause of your problem.

While planning your food, it is good to keep in mind that nature has the ultimate power to heal your health problems and food is the vital medicine you need to adapt as a permanent solution to maintain your vitality and immunity throughout your life. It is good to remember the fact that we humans were treating our health with the essence of nature and had complete trust in those ancient healing sciences until we invented modern medicines a few hundred years back. We still have many medicinal plants that provide us with different vegetables, fruits, herbs, grains, nuts, and beans, but unfortunately we have lost the wisdom of their value or we neglect that information from our ancestors. However, we can return to nature and regain the knowledge to maintain our ultimate health and immunity.

Prior to starting your healthy cooking, you can begin to prepare your natural medicine store, your kitchen, by clearing out your refrigerator. Yes, I mean today. As soon as you stop reading this chapter, go to your kitchen, open your fridge, and look carefully at what you have on those chilled racks. See the inside of your fridge as the inside of your stomach tomorrow, the source of your health and disease. With this image in mind, pull out the unhealthy stuff from your fridge and get rid of it. That is better than it ending up in your stomach, right? Okay, now you can continue your cleaning by searching through your kitchen cupboards, and soon your kitchen and stomach will be clean and tidy, and your body free of future diseases caused by unhealthy food.

Make sure you maintain this level of enthusiasm when you make your next shopping list. Once your kitchen is ready for a health experiment, you can write down or print out the list of foods you want to have in your house and stick it on your fridge or anywhere in the kitchen. You can use the food chart in chapter 11 of this book, or go to my website and print out the latest update of the food list for each dominating force (at janeshvaidya.com/ayurveda/food/).

If you are only preparing food for yourself, you only need to print the food list for your presently dominating force. But if you are making food for your whole family, you can print the food chart for each dominant force (kapha, pitta, and vata). These food lists can help you and your family shop for, prepare, and eat foods according to everyone's dominating elements, which is the best way to maintain optimal health and immune power according to Ayurveda.

With your knowledge of Ayurveda, you can find the right foods for your present mind-body condition. When you find your presently dominating elements with the help of the self-test in chapter 5, you will get to know the leading force in your system at the moment and, according to your PDE, choose the correct natural medicines from your cupboard and start preparing your food.

Perhaps you're wondering how to prepare a dish for your family if they all are different in their PDE. It's a good question, since you need to serve food for all the dominating forces. For example, you might have a pitta domination, your partner kapha, and your children vata. In this situation, I suggest that you use your logic by studying the food list. Some ingredients are appropriate for all dominations, which you can use in general, and the other ingredients that need to be reduced or avoided can be set aside when you start cooking. At different stages of cooking, you can take portions of food out to make sure it is ready to serve for a particular domination. For example, if you are a pitta dominant, before adding strong spices, you can remove your portion of food from the pan and continue adding the ingredients to the rest of the food that is good for the other two dominants, kapha and vata. Other times the spices and the base of the dish might be the same, but you add different vegetables, grains, or beans to the dish according to which domination you are cooking for. This way of preparing food is what I call "smart cooking," because you are using not only your knowledge of Ayurveda but also your logic to make it practical for you as well as healthy for your whole family. This cooking approach has helped many of my clients with family members of different dominations who otherwise would have trouble applying Ayurvedic wisdom in their kitchen.

Cooking is an art, and we can see that many people in this field try to present food in an attractive way by manipulating the essence of the dish, which reduces the quality of nature's medicine. While preparing our food, we need to give our maximum attention to preserve its natural qualities until it reaches our stomach.

Some people have a natural talent for preparing food without using a recipe, and my mother is one of them. I have never seen her follow a recipe or use a measuring cup. All the preparations and quantities are in her brain, and she calculates the amount of each ingredient with her senses.

Preparing a meal is like playing a musical string instrument. For example, the six tastes (sweet, sour, salt, pungent, astringent, and bitter) are like the six strings of a guitar. Just as a musician can play countless pieces of music with a guitar, a talented chef can make an endless number of dishes with the same ingredients by playing with the six tastes. This way we can modify the recipes that are not specifically designed for our dominating elements. By being an artist in our kitchen, we can enjoy the taste of the food with our senses and make each meal a celebration without compromising our health.

In India we consider the kitchen a second prayer room. It has been a practice since ancient times to enter the kitchen in the morning and light the fire in the stove with a silent prayer on the lips. In the kitchen we are not just making food; we are making medicine for our family. And we are not just adding spices to the food, but also our love, which turns into the essential taste of the food we prepare. This must be the reason that people, when they return home to their native countries after doing the Ayurveda treatments in my village, often comment that they have never eaten food as tasty as the food my family served during their stay at the retreat. The secret behind this delicious plant-based food lies not only in the ingredients and the Ayurveda recipes used but also in the way it is prepared in my village, with natural talent and heartfelt dedication.

Though I am not a superb chef, I love cooking my own food. Since I have traveled a lot over the last two decades, spreading the knowledge of Ayurveda around the world, many of my readers and clients wonder how I manage my daily food. Well, it's all about choices. Wherever I travel, my first concern is to find accommodations with a kitchen or at least a pantry. I can compromise and live in a room without furniture, but it's hard for me to live in a place where I don't have the option to cook my own food. But when I don't have any cooking facilities, I find raw food options, picking up organic veggies and sprouts and mixing them in a bowl with a simple salad dressing to include all six tastes. That's it, and it's simple, if we just change the image we have of food from something that is attractive to our eyes, heavy for our stomach, and habitual to our senses (something that we have been eating routinely since our childhood) to something that comes directly from nature and is light and easy for our digestive system, simple and clean for our senses, and fresh and natural in its original form.

Mindful Eating

For some people eating is merely a part of their daily routine, while for others it is a delightful experience. If you want to eat food as your natural medicine and celebrate the experience of each meal, you need to know not only what to eat but also how and when.

How Much Should I Eat to Maintain Good Health?

As a general discipline of Ayurveda, if you are suffering from symptoms of kapha aggravation, such as obesity, asthma, sinusitis, or depression, you need to eat smaller quantities and exclude all kinds of cold food taken directly from the fridge or freezer, like ice cream, which is cold and has fatty properties and can aggravate kapha and its corresponding symptoms.

As we say in my village in India, don't eat until your stomach feels full but rather until you feel that one-third of your stomach is empty. So if you have a kapha aggravation, try to keep one-third of your hunger, instead of eating until you satisfy the last bit of your hunger or even beyond that. And remember not to drink while you are eating, as water can dissolve the digestive acids in the stomach and cause indigestion.

If you have heightened pitta in your system, you need to eat good portions of food each time. A good portion for a pitta dominant is the amount of food that makes that person satisfied but not stuffed. Compared to the other two forces, pitta dominants have the highest levels of acids in their system, and this practice will help their digestive system function smoothly without secreting acids in the digestive channels. In situations where you are suffering from pitta-aggravated issues, such as migraines, hyperacidity, or skin diseases like psoriasis or eczema, you need to eat calming and cooling foods, as listed in the pitta-reducing food chart in chapter 11. Also keep in mind that you should never skip a meal, as this can worsen any problems caused by an excess of pitta that you are already suffering from.

Among your friends or family members, you have probably noticed that some of them can eat a large amount of food without gaining extra weight. This is mainly because of their dominating elements; in this case, they are dominated by the air and ether elements, which control the force of vata. If vata is the dominating force in the body, the challenge is to hydrate the body frequently and to maintain adequate body weight by following the right meal plan with regular eating times. If your digestive system is dominated by the force of vata, the digestive function can be irregular, and considering these variations, you need to adapt your diet accordingly. As a vata dominant, make sure you feed your body with warm, grounding, and oily foods every day.

When Is the Best Time of Day to Eat?

As we have learned, the micro level of our body is made up of the five elements of nature, and our nature is not only inside of our skin but also outside of it. This theory simply states that the seasons and the time of the day influence the functions of our internal organs. So when you know which force is dominating your body, you can maintain the stability of that force by adjusting the time of your meals during the day. Though it may be a bit difficult to understand how the changing of mealtimes can affect your health, since I am following this theory in my own life, I recommend that you try this timetable in your own life and feel the difference in your digestion and metabolism in the coming weeks.

With the help of the PDE test in chapter 5, if you find that your dominating force is kapha, you need to avoid eating during the kapha-aggravating time in the nature, which is early morning, from 4:00 a.m. to 10:00 a.m. For instance, if you are suffering from any of the kapha symptoms, particularly obesity, you shouldn't give your body a single chance to gain more weight, right? So don't eat during the time of the day when kapha is more prominent. Instead, eat a light breakfast at 10:00 a.m. and let your lunch be your first regular meal of the day. Drink water or tea in the morning to cleanse your system of the toxic substances that have accumulated in the body. Try this practice for three weeks and note the difference in your health and vitality by balancing your excess kapha.

However, if you are a pitta dominant, don't even think about the previous idea. In this case, the very first thing you need to think about in the morning is your delicious breakfast. I can see the smile on your face if you already took the test and determined that your dominating force is pitta. Yes, you need to eat several times a day, and the main thing to keep in mind is to eat calming and cooling foods, especially in the middle of the day, when the energy of the sun is at its peak, especially on a hot summer day. If you are not careful with pitta-aggravating food, it can easily trigger your pitta-related symptoms, such as acidity issues in the body and stress in the mind, especially in hot climates and in the middle of the day.

If you live far from the equator, you can consider the evening as the vata-aggravating time of day. If you are a vata dominant, you need to eat warm and grounding food in the evening as your dinner, especially when the temperature outside is less than 20 degrees Celsius (68 Fahrenheit). Considering the state of your digestion, make sure to get the right spices through your food, which will help to pacify your vata and reduce the air-ether imbalance symptoms, such as joint pain in the body and anxiety in the mind. The vata-balancing food you eat in the evening will stay in your stomach like a warm blanket throughout the night and promote better sleep.

How to Eat Mindfully

When I first arrived in Europe, one of the most surprising things I noticed was that many people have the ability to talk continuously while they are eating with other people. This strange practice seems to be a part of socializing, especially in the more industrially developed countries. I still don't know how they manage this shuffling technique inside the mouth without the words and the food colliding with each other. Unfortunately, this ability (or disability!) destroys the essence of mindful eating. This must be the reason many people in the West avoid booking lunch meetings with me, because they have noticed that I don't have the ability to talk while I am eating. The moment the dish arrives in front of me, I forget everything around me but the food.

There is an old saying in my village: drink your food and eat your water. Though it sounds funny, if we think about the logic behind it, we can understand what it actually means. Our food has three layers of taste, and when we eat in a hurry, we only connect with the first layer and miss the two layers underneath. While the first layer of taste is connected to our taste buds on the tongue, the other subtle layers are connected to our consciousness, which we can sense only through a mindful eating practice.

To practice mindful eating, I suggest that you do the following:

1. Before you begin to eat, take three deep breaths with your eyes closed, and make your mind calm and your body relaxed.

2. Be grateful and say thanks to the universe for this plate of food in front of you.

3. Imagine the taste of your food by pausing any other thoughts inside your brain.

4. Always try to sit and eat in your own space of silence.

5. During eating times, don't encourage other people to talk by giving them your attention or eye contact. (Keep your eyes focused on your plate of food.)

6. Chew your food around 14 to 25 times and drink your food.

7. By melting each bit of food in your mouth, enjoy it with complete satisfaction.

8. Avoid thoughts that try to enter your mind while chewing, especially thoughts that create anger, sadness, or worry.

9. Never hurry to finish your meal, and stay in that feeling of satisfaction to prolong the delicious moment.

Since childhood, it has been a natural practice for me to sit in front of my meal for a few seconds of silence. It is a part of our custom to say a silent prayer before starting each meal. The purpose of all these rituals is to give the food the proper respect and our body enough time, and to draw the focus of our mind to our plate of food, even before we bring nature's healing properties into our body.

When we eat in silence, with the utmost focus, we can sense the deeper layers of taste in each molecule of food. We can feel the melting point of each bit of nature's essence on our tongue before we drink our food. You can experience the art of eating when you meditate with your food.

How Many Times a Day Can a Person Eat?

Usually two to three hours are required for the first part of the digestion process of a natural food, and a person can eat half a palmful (of chewed food) three to five times a day. As I have mentioned, this varies from person to person and from time to time according to the PDE.

The consumption of food also depends on the physical activities of a person, so the required nutritional values and the frequency of food intake have to be designed with consideration for the lifestyle-influencing factors. But the habit of eating small quantities of high-quality food will definitely make a difference in your metabolism. Through this practice, you can feel good energy in your body and enthusiasm in your mind, and keep a good immune power and vitality so you can stay healthy throughout the days and different seasons.

How Can I Improve My Digestion?

One of the important disciplines I would like to share from my own experience is to have different times for eating and drinking. As we say in my village, don't drink while eating and don't eat while drinking. This yogic practice helps you maintain a powerful digestion and a strong stomach.

When you eat your main meals, like lunch or dinner, your stomach needs to have enough agni (digestive fire) to absorb the nourishment from your food. If you drink before, during, or after your meal, this digestive fire is subdued and the body has less power to break down the food molecules in the stomach, and this causes slow digestion or indigestion. To avoid this situation and improve your digestive fire, Ayurveda suggests taking a break from drinking at least half an hour before your main meals and waiting for at least one hour after a meal to take your next drink. This also allows you to focus more on your food and prevents you from swallowing the food before it is properly chewed. Remember that the status of your stomach is the first sign of your health.

I also recommend practicing *vajrasana* (diamond pose) for three to seven minutes after your main meals, which supports better bowel movements and digestion. (Diamond pose: Sit on a mat on the floor in a kneeling position. Rest your hands on your thighs and lengthen your spine.)

Celebrate Each Meal!

In the villages in India, you often see people singing and dancing after they have had a delicious meal. Yes, you can make these people the happiest merely by serving them a good meal! But I wonder how many people in the West would be this happy only because of getting a good meal?

From now on, take the matter of food seriously and look forward to your coming meals of the day. And at the end of each day, dream of the coming days' delightful meals. I know what you are thinking right now: how can we find time in our busy day to think about or plan our food properly? Well, how about if we save enough time for the most important practices in our life, like making food, love, and laughter? Otherwise we miss the essence of this beautiful life on this wonderful planet. To find enough time, we need to prioritize food as one of the first preferences on our list by saving time for it, instead of spending time on less important matters such as social media or involving ourselves in matters in other people's lives that are not directly connected with us and our health.

Ayurveda Guidelines for Eating

- Eat at regular times.
- Drink warm water or herbal tea during the day.
- Avoid drinking with meals.

- Chew your drink and drink your food.
- Allow enough time between meals to fully digest the previous meal.
- Avoid fast food.
- Shop, cook, and eat consciously.
- Use spices (the right ones for your PDE).
- Eat food with clean energy (plant-based).
- Eat home-cooked food.
- Eat in a calm environment.
- Sit down when eating.
- Make eating your meditation.

These are general guidelines to improve the quality of your food disciplines. In the coming chapters you will find specific advice based on your presently dominating elements.

Chapter 7

FIVE-STAGE PLAN TO BUILD OPTIMAL RESISTANCE POWER

Before we get into the discussion about personalized diet plans in the coming sections, I want to give you an overview of the different stages of your health and immunity that you will pass through while you adapt food as your natural medicine and follow the Ayurveda recommendations according to your presently dominating elements. With the help of the chart at the beginning of this chapter, you get an outline of how you can change your health for the better. By following the five-stage meal plan, you can ease the symptoms you might be suffering from at present. To get an overview, I have laid out a chart that shows the gradual changes in your internal system after 21 days, 3 months, 6 months, and beyond when you work on your health by creating healthy habits with your best plant-based food. In the next few chapters you will gain knowledge of the medicinal properties of each force and the correlation with the six tastes of food according to the principles of Ayurveda. This wisdom will help you understand the role of natural food in improving your health and the Ayurvedic way of self-healing.

Over the last two decades of my practice and research in the field of plant-based food around the world, I have implemented a five-stage health improvement program, with which I have been treating my clients in their healing process of various health issues. Considering that every meal plays an important role in rebuilding (or destroying) our health, it is essential to know the right foods for your PDE (presently dominating elements) and monitor their effects on your health through the five stages of the food program.

Imagine that today is the first day of your life and your health, for the rest of your life depends on what you eat and not eat from now on. Keep the mantra in your mind that food is your natural medicine and health is your conscious choice.

My new clients often ask me what foods or drinks they have to add to their daily meal plan to achieve better health. I often remind them that instead of pondering what you have to eat, think about what you shouldn't eat. Nowadays many people in our society get sick not because of a lack of food, but because of an excess of unhealthy food that creates ama (toxins) and blocks the system's natural function and eventually leads to disease. So, as an initial step in your five-stage health improvement program, I suggest that you identify your unhealthy food and drink habits and swap them for healthy habits.

In the chart here, the numbers will vary slightly according to the number of days in every month; each month is calculated as thirty days for a general estimate of the meals.

Stage 1: First 21 Days

The first twenty-one days of the food practice is the biggest challenge for most people who want to improve their health by changing old, unhealthy habits into new, healthy habits. But once you have managed the first three weeks of your new food plan, your body will have received a minimum of 63 rejuvenating meals (calculated as three main meals per day—breakfast, lunch, and dinner). Consider this to be one of the most important challenges of your life to regain your natural health. Throughout the entire journey, try to stick to your healthy food choices without letting outside voices and old habits distract your senses and weaken your determination.

Five-Stage Health Improvement Program

Stage	Duration of Stage	Number of Meals	Health Benefits
1	First 21 days	63 meals	Your habits change into health—a sign of your determination.
2	Days 22–90	+ 207 meals	Your stomach functions happily—the first sign of your health improvement.
3	Days 91–180	+ 270 meals	Your body pain and inflammation are eliminated—the body's first level cleansing of old toxins.
4	Day 181 through year 2	+ 1,620 meals	Your symptoms disappear—a sign that your body has started its natural healing process.
5	Year 3 through year 7	+ 5,400 meals	Your body is reaching Kakajanmam*—a sign that a major part of your old body cells have been replaced with new, healthy cells after seven years of practicing your personal diet according to your PDE.

Kakajanmam: According to the traditional belief in Ayurveda, during a seven-year period, a human body replaces a major part of its cells. If you take care of your health with the right food disciplines, within seven years you can refresh your body systems and restart your life as a newborn, with more youthfulness and vitality. This seven-year cleansing and rejuvenation program not only relieves the body of symptoms and diseases but also reverses the aging process of the person who passes through these five stages.

Stage 2: Day 22 Through Day 90

When you finish this stage of the challenge three months after the start of the program, your body will have received approximately 270 (63 + 207) rejuvenating meals. During these three months, with the healing power of the Ayurveda food for your PDE, you will see the first signs of health in your body, which manifests as a happy, well-functioning stomach. By the end of this stage, you may feel that your digestive system is performing better than ever.

Stage 3: Day 91 Through Day 180

During the third stage of the plan, with the help of your personal diet, your body eliminates the old toxins that have accumulated in your system. As per the calculation of three main meals a day, during the six months since you started the program, your body will have received around 540 (63 + 207 + 270) rejuvenating meals for your PDE, which cleanse the channels and improve the functions of the circulatory system in the body.

Stage 4: Day 181 Through Year 2

The cleansing and healing process continues during the fourth stage of the food plan, which lasts up to two years from the start of the program and includes approximately 2,160 (63 + 207 + 270 + 1,620) rejuvenating meals for your PDE. During this period, most of your long-term symptoms disappear and you regain the vitality of your body and the focus and clarity of your mind.

Stage 5: Year 3 Through Year 7

When you enter the fifth stage of the program, your challenge becomes your best friend and encourages you to take on even more healthy habits in the future with the support of the results you experienced during the last couple of years. According to this five-stage health improvement program, in a total of seven years your body will have received around 7,560 rejuvenating meals (63 + 207 + 270 + 1,620 + 5,400), and most of the old cells in your body will have been replaced with new cells, created with the essence of the healing food and drink you ingested during this period. By this time you will feel like a newborn, with a vigorous body and a clear mind, which we call *kaka-janmam* in the traditional Ayurveda practice in South India.

See this five-stage rejuvenating plan as a train stopping at five stations, showing the health results you will experience through the coming days. Instead of postponing your journey until the next day, get up on the health train and start the program now, and look out the window from the inside of the moving car, counting down the days and months and years with the progress in your health calendar.

Keep in mind that your PDE might change during the course of your program, especially if you have a vikruti in any of the three forces in your mind-body system at the beginning of your program. So I suggest that you take the PDE self-test in chapter 5 after each stage of the program until you enter the fourth stage, and then do the test every three months to make sure you are following the right diet plan for your PDE. Once your elements are balanced with this program, you will get your PDE result as your prakruti, which will remain unchanged, and your body and mind will stay in a state of optimal health and immunity as long as you follow the Ayurveda recommendations in your daily life.

To start the five-stage health improvement program, first find your PDE with the help of the "Find Your Imbalance" test in chapter 5. Then determine the right foods for you (vegetables, fruits, grains, nuts, seeds, legumes, etc.) using the food chart in chapter 11. To find recipes for your PDE, you can refer to my cookbooks or follow the recipes on my website, which will not only help you design a healthy meal plan but also open up the world for your taste buds to the symphony of the six tastes from the Ayurveda cuisine.

Chapter 8

THE FOOD THAT BOOSTS YOUR IMMUNE POWER

In this chapter you will become acquainted with the six tastes of Ayurveda and their correlation to the food that promotes health and immunity. By understanding how the constitutional elements of the six rasas (tastes) influence the three forces of our body and mind, we can choose the right food and eat according to the present condition of our body. When we recognize our food through the six tastes, we become our own therapist, using nature's natural healing properties in our diet to promote balance and health instead of imbalance and disease in our systems.

Apart from us humans, all other species on the planet naturally use food as their only medicine to maintain their health. And they gain this wisdom directly from nature and practice it throughout their lives with their senses, while we humans are busy trying to collect information from the literature and struggling to practice inside our square rooms. If we can trust Mother Nature and treat her with respect, the healing process will begin in our life, too, with signs of health, inside and out.

The Six Rasas (Tastes)

To understand the use of food as medicine, Ayurveda defines food as nature's essence that is recognized by its six tastes, which are sweet, sour, salt, pungent, bitter, and astringent. Whether it is a fruit or a vegetable, a nut or a grain, the properties of each food item vary according to the dominating elements in it, which we can sense by its natural taste. When you eat food with a particular taste, remember that its effect on your body is determined by the property of that food.

For example, foods and drinks with the taste of sweet and salt are highly dominated by the earth and water elements, and when we eat food with these tastes, it will naturally increase the force of kapha in our system. Kapha-property food supports the body by generating new tissues and is used as a medicine when the force of vata is high in the system, as vata is a destructive force for the tissues and strongly influences the body during old age and in cold seasons.

All foods and drinks with the tastes of sour and pungent are highly dominated by the fire and water elements, and the intake of food items with these tastes can boost the force of pitta in the system. Pitta-property food controls the digestive and circulatory systems, maintaining the body temperature and thus the immune power.

Foods that taste bitter or astringent have vata-increasing properties because of the domination of the air and either elements in them. Most Ayurveda medicines are bitter and astringent in their basic taste and have medicinal properties that can eliminate toxins in the system.

To improve your health with nature's medicinal plants, grains, beans, nuts, seeds, fruits, and vegetables, you can learn more about the six tastes and make use of their properties in your daily meal plan according to your PDE (presently dominating elements).

Sweet

In nature, everything we sense as sweet is a sign of attraction and connection, embedded in every flower and fruit to fulfill the purpose of reproduction. While the proper use of natural sweet provides self-confidence, satisfaction, and happiness, overuse can generate strong demands and attachments in our relationships. Sweet is essential to maintain healthy tissues in the body, but in excess it creates congestion in our systems and leads to being overweight, and in later stages causes diseases of the organs. Overuse of sweet over a long period of time, especially the concentrated sweets available in stores, can impair the functions of the pancreas and spleen.

Since we need starchy food to generate new cells in the body, the lack of sweet in our diet can lead to malnutrition. Most grains are sweet in their basic taste and a natural source of starchy food. They are cold in their properties and increase kapha but reduce pitta and stabilize vata. Therefore, I have designed the kapha-reducing recipes for my guests at the retreat in my village in India with less starch and fewer sweet ingredients. The earth and water elements in the sweet and starchy foods nourish the body tissues and help the natural process of growth, which is favorable for pitta and vata dominants.

Nowadays one of the biggest threats to our health is the overuse of sweets. Concentrated sugar is a common ingredient in most of the food supplied in stores, and according to Ayurveda, sugar is considered to be a white poison. Make sure you use the sweet taste only from natural sources (not concentrated or processed ones) and according to your current dominant elements.

Sour

Sour is the natural supplier of acid, the liquid form of fire aiding the digestive system, which is essential to maintain healthy digestion and metabolism. However, sour is harmful to the organs if the acid in the system exceeds a certain limit, as if the fire in the kitchen got out of control.

In our human body, we normally consider the optimal state of the pH level of the blood to be between 7.30 to 7.45; we can say somewhat above 7. This is where acid and alkaline come into equilibrium. If the pH level goes below the neutral state of 7, it means the acidity level is higher in our body, which increases the level of agni, the fire element, and aggravates the force of pitta, causing damage to the digestive system, especially in the liver and gallbladder. The physical symptoms can appear as psoriasis, eczema, or migraine, for example, and can lead to tumors in the long run. If the acidity is high in the body systems, it can also affect us mentally; we may feel high stress levels and become egoistic in relationships. On the other hand, if the pH level rises (low acidity) in the body over a long period and reaches a very high alkaline level, it can lead to indigestion.

Please do keep in mind that some food items can be exceptions to this modern acid-alkaline theory. For example, although lemon is sour in its basic property, after being processed in the stomach it changes its property to alkaline. Lime, unripened orange, and grape are also sour fruits in their prime property, but after digestion they turn alkaline. And some food items (for example, white rice) are not acidic in their prime property, but after processing in the stomach they become acidic.

Ayurveda considers the properties of each food in terms of its effect on the body in three stages: rasa, virya, and vipaka. While rasa is the primary property of food from nature, sensed by our taste glands as sweet, sour, salt, pungent, bitter, or astringent, virya is the overall effect of that food on the body (cooling or heating), and vipaka is the bio-transformative phase of rasa, which happens after the digestion of the food in the stomach. In Ayurveda food recipes, the main concern is the prime property (rasa), which is the property of the food until it reaches the inside of the stomach. That is why sour fruits are categorized as digestion-aiding acids, promoting the liquid form of fire in the stomach. Most Ayurvedic plant-based food is alkaline in its virya and vipaka stages, even though some are acidic in the rasa stage until they are digested.

It is good to remember that the effect of a food on the body also changes according to natural transformations. Acidic fruits, such as citrus, and fermented food and vinegar fall in this category. Most fruits are sour in the beginning, become sweet when they ripen, and turn to sour again through the fermentation process. Young grapes, for example, are sour, then they grow into sweet grapes, and then, through a fermentation process, they turn into wine, which is both sour and sweet in its properties.

Although sour boosts all the functions of the tissues, overuse of this taste can decrease the function of the reproductive glands. This is one reason I usually recommend reducing the use of sour in the diet for people who lack sexual drive. Sour is hot in its character and greatly increases pitta. It also increases kapha but reduces the vata force.

Salt

Salt is one of the most essential tastes for a smooth function of the joints and intestines. A salt deficiency can lead to constipation and stiffness in the body and a negative attitude in the mind. Though the earth and fire elements of salt work as a laxative to support the digestive system, excessive use of salt over a long period can impair the functions of the kidneys and adrenal glands. Overuse of salt can also increase the blood pressure and affect the heart function. Mentally, this taste in excess can generate greediness and dissatisfaction in life.

When I design individual diets for the guests in my village, I sometimes recommend adding iodized sea salt to the food, since iodine is one of the essential trace minerals for the function of two thyroid hormones, thyroxine (T4) and triiodothyronine (T3). But it is important to know how much iodine you need per day, which is determined according to your PDE and other factors.

The basic property of salt is moist, oily, heavy, and hot, and it can increase pitta and kapha but it reduces vata. Though salt is a digestive aid, if we use it in excess, it can cause nausea and vomiting. In Ayurveda treatments, salt has a special role, especially in internal cleansing treatments.

Pungent

South Indian people are known for their fondness for spicy food, and it has been quite hard to train the local chefs at my health retreat in Kerala to prepare food for my guests without making it too spicy. I often remind them that, as with the sour taste, the prime property of pungent is fire, which needs to be controlled in the food. Otherwise the mind can get disturbed with anger and frustration, and in the long run generate negative emotions such as hatred. At the same time, the absence of the pungent taste can slow down the digestion and reduce the level of enthusiasm in the mind.

Since agni, the fire element, is one of the major factors maintaining the immune system through the digestion and metabolism in the body, we need to keep the right amount of spices in our daily diet according to the level of our PDE (presently dominating elements). While a lack of pungent properties in the diet can cause indigestion and slow bowel movements, excessive use of this taste can lead to symptoms such as hyperacidity and acid reflux.

Pungent increases pitta and vata but reduces the force of kapha. The fire and air elements of the pungent taste aid the digestion and metabolism by promoting the digestive fire in the system and regulating the temperature of the body by releasing water as sweat. A moderate use of pungent supports the function of the lymphatic and digestive systems.

Bitter

In my early years, when I got my first lessons from my grandma, she taught me how to recognize medicinal plants through my senses, especially by their taste. In those days I noticed that most medicinal plants were bitter in their basic taste. Bitter has the highest medicinal value, followed by astringent and pungent. In my village, we use the leaves with the most bitter properties for the Ayurveda treatments, considering their natural healing properties, and they are the base of medicines for different illnesses.

The bitter taste has the opposite qualities of the sweet taste, and it detoxifies our body by purifying the blood and removing ama (toxins) that has accumulated in the system. With their cooling and dehydrating properties, the air and ether elements of bitter increase vata but decrease pitta and kapha. Through the elimination of excess fat in our internal channels, bitter promotes better blood circulation to the cells, maintaining maximum immune power on the micro level of the body.

Most alkaline foods have a bitter and astringent taste. Though bitter is high in medicinal properties, overuse of this taste in food, without consideration of the dominating element and season, can slow down the function of the heart and awaken sadness and depression. That is one reason I suggest reducing bitter vegetables for vata dominant clients, especially in the winter season, when vata has a strong effect in nature.

Since bitter is a natural detoxifier, there is nothing better than to add this taste to the daily diet of those who want to reduce excess weight and toxins, especially the kapha dominants. I also add bitter to the diet of patients carrying self-hatred, which can be eliminated by using this natural detoxifying taste.

Astringent

Astringent is an anti-inflammatory medicine for the body tissues. To reduce inflammation in the body, I recommend that you add the astringent taste to your daily diet (with consideration of your PDE). However, overuse of this natural anti-inflammatory medicine in your diet can disturb the functions of the intestines and rectum and generate fear and nervousness in the mind.

Most vegetables and plant-based foods contain medicinal properties, which we can recognize through the bitter and astringent tastes. Like the bitter taste, the cooling and drying properties of astringent decrease pitta and kapha, respectively, but increase vata. The anti-inflammatory properties of the earth and air elements in the astringent taste work in the body to eliminate excess water, which can lead to inflammation and pain if the fluid accumulates and stays in the tissues for a long time.

The astringent taste also protects the body from dehydration and excess discharges such as heavy sweating and bleeding, especially during menstruation or a wound-healing process. For instance, all plants with strong healing properties of astringent and bitter, such as aloe vera, can be used to heal external or internal wounds in the body and prevent infection.

The Influence of the Six Tastes on the Three Forces

From now on, see the food you eat through your tongue, and sense its medicinal effects with your taste buds. That simply means understand the six tastes of food and their effects on your health according to the application of these tastes in your daily food. For example, if you are a kapha dominant at present and are suffering from symptoms of excess kapha in your system, you know which of the six tastes to avoid and which to add to your diet. In the following chart, you can see that sweet and salt highly increase kapha, as does sour to a certain extent. At the same time, bitter food highly reduces kapha, and the astringent and pungent tastes do as well to a certain extent. This means that you should avoid the sweet and salt tastes and use sour only at a moderate level, but add the bitter taste in a high proportion and use the astringent and pungent tastes frequently in your daily food. Likewise, if you have an aggravation in pitta or vata and are suffering from the corresponding symptoms, you can follow the recommendations in the chart to increase or decrease certain tastes. If you try to follow this theory in your daily diet, you will see health improvements reflected in a better-functioning digestive system and increased immune power.

In the following chart, the symbols minus (−), minus minus (− −), plus (+), and plus plus (+ +) are used to show how much each taste affects each force according to its food properties.

The Effects of the Six Tastes on the Three Forces

Rasa (Taste)	Vata	Pitta	Kapha
Sweet	−	− −	+ +
Sour	−	+ +	+
Salt	−	+	+ +
Pungent (spicy)	+	+ +	−
Bitter	+	−	− −
Astringent	+ +	−	−
Key:			
−	decreases the force to a minimum degree		
− −	decreases the force to a maximum degree		
+	increases the force to a minimum degree		
++	increases the force to a maximum degree		

The Effects of the Six Tastes on Our Body and Mind Functions

In the next two charts, we can see which effects we may experience on our body and mind due to an excess or a lack of each taste. These charts are for general use, but if you have any physical or mental symptoms at the moment, you can use this information to reduce the use of the rasa (taste) that is irritating your health and instead add the rasa that can decrease your symptoms. For example, if you have an issue with acidity that is disturbing the function of your stomach or esophagus, try to avoid or reduce the use of the pungent taste by being careful with spicy food. If you apply this Ayurveda theory to your diet for a few days or weeks, you will see improvements in the function of your corresponding organs and positive changes in your mental status.

While the first chart here lists the effects of an excessive use of each taste (rasa) in your food, the second chart lists the physical and mental issues caused by a lack of each taste in the diet.

If you are suffering from any of the issues listed in these charts, eliminate or add the corresponding taste that can defuse or improve your health issue. But remember to take small steps by eliminating or adding rasas a little at a time, so as not to upset your stomach and mind.

The Effects of an Excessive Use of the Six Tastes in Your Food

Excess of Taste (+ +)	Damage in the Body	Feelings and Emotions in the Mind
Sweet	Pancreas and spleen	Demands and attachment in love
Sour	Liver and bile	Ego and jealousy
Salt	Kidneys and adrenal glands	Greed and dissatisfaction
Pungent	Stomach and esophagus	Anger and hate
Bitter	Heart and veins	Sadness and depression
Astringent	Intestines and rectum	Nervousness and fear

The Effects of a Deficiency of the Six Tastes in Your Food

Deficiency of Taste (– –)	Effects on the Body	Effects on the Mind
Sweet	Malnutrition	Lack of self-confidence
Sour	Gas formation	Inferiority complex
Salt	Constipation, stiffness in the muscles	Negative attitude
Pungent	Slow digestion	Less enthusiastic
Bitter	Toxin, fat accumulation, obesity	Self-hatred, suicidal
Astringent	Pain and inflammation	Deep anxiety

STRENGTHEN YOUR IMMUNITY WITH THE MEDICINAL PROPERTIES OF THE ELEMENTS

After learning about the effects of the different rasas (the different tastes of food) on our body and mind, we now move on to examine the medicinal properties of food and their role in balancing the elements and thus pacifying the forces in our system. In this chapter you will learn more about the therapeutic value of the five elements and their healing powers in your system, according to your presently dominating elements (PDE).

· · · · · · · · · · · · ·

Let us begin by studying the properties of different foods according to their dominating elements and how they can increase the level of the forces in our system. As with our body cells, each food item, whether it is a vegetable or a fruit, a grain or a nut, contains on the micro level the properties of the five natural elements: earth, water, fire, air, and ether. And as in our body, even though all five elements are present in all foods, every food item is dominated by a certain combination of elements. When we eat an item of food, it increases the level of the corresponding elements and decreases the level of the opposite elements in our body, and hence the corresponding force is increased and the opposite force is decreased.

When you recognize foods through the basic characteristics of their dominating elements, you can correct the disorders in your system by choosing food with the properties opposite to those of the elements that are high in your system. For example, if you have an aggravation in the vata force (caused by excess of the air and ether elements), you can use kapha-increasing food (earth and water elements) as medicine to reduce your vata, and vice versa if you have a kapha aggravation. According to this theory, an avocado is a medicine for vata because it has properties that are grounding, heavy, fatty, and nourishing, which increases kapha but reduces vata. Here you can see that the same fruit has a double effect: while it increases kapha, it reduces vata. If you learn how to use the properties of each food for different ailments, you will become a pharmacist by transforming your kitchen into your own medical store, where you prepare the daily medicine for yourself and your family with the essence of nature, with the wisdom of Ayurveda.

A detailed study of the therapeutic qualities of each element can help you treat the ailments of the body by using the properties of one element against the other imbalanced element. This is one of the most practical ways to learn about nature's five elements and three forces and to sustain your and your family's health. To get a deeper understanding, first we can look at the characteristics of the three forces formed by the five elements, and their similarities and differences, shown in the following chart.

Characteristics of the Three Forces

Vata	Cold	Light	Dry
Pitta	Hot	Light	Moist
Kapha	Cold	Heavy	Moist

Medicinal Food Properties of the Earth and Water Elements (Kapha)

When old cells are destroyed by the force of vata, new cells are generated and replaced by the force of kapha by receiving nourishment from the food. Hence our body grows with the force of kapha, formed by the earth and water elements.

Food dominated by earth and water has grounding and cooling properties, such as food rich in carbohydrates and essential fats. Most nuts, beans, and grains have these kapha-increasing properties and support the body to generate new tissues and the process of growth.

Kapha-increasing food is good to pacify the other two forces, such as when excess heat is generated by the aggravated force of pitta, or to control the force of vata in situations where the air and ether elements are making the body too fragile and the mind ungrounded. But if we don't control the food rich in the earth and water elements in our diet, it can cause obesity and related symptoms by increasing body mass and creating a dull and depressed mind. This means that even though kapha-boosting food has medicinal properties, if we don't regulate the use of this food in our diet according to our present health condition, it can also cause problems with its earth- and water-increasing effects.

People who are overweight, as well as those suffering from heart diseases, asthma, or bronchitis, need to reduce kapha-increasing food to improve function of the circulatory and respiratory systems.

Keep in mind that food that is sweet, heavy, oily, and cold in nature is kapha-aggravating.

Let's take a closer look at the three most important medicinal properties of food rich in the earth and water elements.

1. Lubricating

Properties: Oily, fat, and lubricating

Examples: Avocado, nuts with a high fat content

Benefits: Maintains the elasticity of the skin and the lubrication of the internal systems

The Ayurveda perspective: With an excess of vata, the air element dries out the moist oil content in the system, which causes extra dryness in the body tissues. The lack of fatty acids also slows down the function of the sebaceous glands and causes dryness of the skin, hair, and nails, which eventually become fragile and show signs of early aging. Excess vata also makes young skin hard and wrinkly in the absence of oil in the food. To pacify the aggravated vata and to avoid dryness and internal pain caused by a lack of lubrication in the system, it is essential to add oily kapha-increasing food to the diet.

2. Cooling

Properties: Calming, saturated, and cold

Example: Coconut oil

Benefits: Gives solidity and has a cooling and calming effect

The Ayurveda perspective: Kapha-increasing food is most essential in situations of increased vata and pitta on the body level or aggravated pitta on the mind level. Food with the earth and water elements is favorable for people who are suffering from less body weight, but keep in mind that when treating vata with cooling kapha-increasing food, the food has to be heated to counteract its cold properties; otherwise it can aggravate vata as an aftereffect. The proper use of the earth and water elements in food can enhance mental qualities such as patience and stability and help reduce stress.

3. Nourishing

Properties: Sweet, heavy, grounding, and nourishing

Examples: Rice, sweet potato

Benefits: Generates new cells and reduces oxidization

The Ayurveda perspective: If we don't nourish our body in a timely fashion with food that is rich in the earth and water elements, it will lead to rapid aging of the internal and external organs. (The vata force destroys cells to support the aging process.) For example, a human body usually loses an average of 50 to 130 hairs each day with the function of vata, so to maintain the same amount of hair, the system has to be nourished with the properties of the earth and water elements. If the body shows signs of high vata or pitta, it releases more hair than normal, and if these issues are not rectified with kapha-increasing food, the density of the hair will decrease over time. This is the same condition that occurs with the destruction and generation of skin cells and all the other tissues in the body. A deficiency of the earth and water elements in the system also causes problems in the mind, such as a lack of concentration, sleep disturbances, ungrounded feelings, deep anxiety, and stress. To avoid these symptoms in situations of hyper pitta and hyper vata in the body and mind, be sure to maintain a rich variety of kapha-increasing food in your diet. However, in a state of aggravated kapha, try to avoid or reduce food that increases the earth and water elements, especially in situations where the other two forces (pitta and vata) are very low in the system.

Medicinal Food Properties of the Fire and Water Elements (Pitta)

Pitta-increasing food is moist, light, and/or hot in its basic properties and maintains the agni (fire) in the digestive system. Most spices fall into this category. The proper level of these digestive aids in the food can promote a better metabolism and immune power.

Food high in the fire and water elements is useful in situations of excess kapha or low vata, where the acidic property of the food supports the digestion and balances the elements that control the corresponding forces. But if pitta is already high in the system, such a diet can cause acidity and related symptoms.

Our stomach is the kitchen of our body, and the acids and enzymes in our digestive system act as the fire required to prepare the food in the kitchen. If the fire rises too high in the kitchen and gets out of control, what will happen? The flames could burn down the entire house. The same applies if the fire element in our body exceeds its limits. With the excess heat, our organs develop problems. For instance, in the state of pitta aggravation, the largest organ of our body, our skin, can get eczema or psoriasis, our food channels can have problems with acidity and acid reflux, and many other physical and mental symptoms can be caused by the excess of acid in the system. So let me ask you: if you had a fire in your house, would you pour water or gas on it to extinguish the flames?

We all need a balanced level of the fire element in our system to maintain good health and immunity through proper digestion and metabolism. Keeping this in mind, we need to use the right amount of pitta-increasing food in our diet according to our present health condition. When we have slow digestion in the absence of enough fire in the system, we need to add pitta-increasing food, and when we suffer from hyperacidity in our digestive system and its negative effects on our body and mind, we need to reduce or even eliminate foods that have the potential to increase the force of pitta.

Let's take a closer look at the three most important medicinal properties of food rich in the fire and water elements.

1. Digestive

Properties: Hot and acidic

Examples: Pepper, ginger, lemon

Benefits: Supports the digestion

The Ayurveda perspective: Pitta-increasing food is hot and acidic in its basic properties. Like a fire in the kitchen, the pitta properties manifest as digestive acids and enzymes on the tongue and in the stomach, pancreas, liver, and small intestines to support the digestion. In a cold atmosphere, vata and kapha dominants are recommended to maintain a diet rich in fire and water to counteract the low temperature. However, in a warm atmosphere, pitta dominants have to take extra care to avoid pitta-boosting food, which can irritate the agni in the blood and manifest as various skin disorders. Hence, it is essential to take the climate and the seasons into consideration when designing your diet.

People with digestion problems such as constipation or diarrhea need to avoid pitta-increasing food and drink, since they can worsen those conditions. Pitta dominants usually suffer from hyperacidity in the stomach and dehydration in the colon, the result of excess heat and acids in the digestive system. If this situation continues over a long time, it can cause stomach ulcers and piles. At the same time, kapha dominants tend to have slow digestion (manda agni), which needs to be rectified with food dominated by the water and fire elements.

2. Antibacterial

Properties: Sour, moist, and acidic

Examples: Citrus fruits and grapes

Benefit: Protects skin from bacterial infections

The Ayurveda perspective: The quality of the skin changes according to the dominant elements. For example, dehydration can be high in a body dominated by air and ether, but less in a system dominated by earth and water. That is one of the primary reasons Ayurveda recommends that vata dominants consume kapha- and pitta-increasing foods to maintain the elasticity of the skin.

Many natural skin products contain spices and fruits with antibacterial qualities. With the help of pitta, the sebaceous glands in the body produce sebum, which protects the skin from external infections. Sebum contains acids and oil. While the acidic property protects the skin from bacterial infections, the oil maintains the elasticity of the skin. In our modern life, the use of chemical shampoos and soaps often washes away the natural moisture of the sebum, causing extra dryness and fast aging of the skin.

3. Cardiac Aid

Properties: Spicy, thinning, and light

Examples: Chili, black pepper, raw onion

Benefits: Decreases cholesterol and improves cardiac health

The Ayurveda perspective: Foods that boost pitta and vata are recommended for kapha dominants because of their light and thinning qualities. This helps people with a kapha domination to melt the fat molecules in the bloodstream and regulate high blood pressure and cholesterol, which increases the health and life span of the circulatory system. However, overuse of pitta-aggravating food (especially for a pitta dominant) will increase the acidity level in the blood. Because of the excess heat, the blood becomes thinner and the blood pressure often drops to the lowest levels, reducing the power of the immune cells in the blood. This is one reason that pitta dominants are often prone to infection compared to the other two dominants.

Medicinal Food Properties of the
Air and Ether Elements (Vata)

The force of vata shares one physical property with pitta (light) and one with kapha (cold). So when we use food with air and ether properties to pacify aggravated pitta or kapha, our focus should be on the properties that are opposite to those of the disturbed force.

Food with properties of the air and ether elements is bitter and astringent in its basic taste. While the bitter taste is a detoxifier, the astringent acts as an anti-inflammatory agent in the body. Vata-increasing food is dry, light, and cold in its physical qualities. While the first two qualities pacify kapha, the first and third qualities pacify pitta.

To practice Ayurveda in life, it is essential to know the properties of each food type in order to treat or prevent symptoms. The logic behind it is that if one force is out of balance, use the force (or forces) that is opposite to it and let those properties counteract it.

The use of anti-inflammatory and detoxifying food with air and ether properties (with an awareness of your presently dominating elements) works as a medicine to eliminate inflammation and toxins in the body.

Our body systems require the timely cleansing of ama (toxins) from the air, water, and food we consume in our everyday life. Most plants and vegetables have the power to absorb inflammation from the muscles and joint tissues and to clear the toxic content from the channels.

Let's take a closer look at the three most important medicinal properties of food rich in the air and ether elements.

1. Anti-inflammatory

Properties: Bitter, dry, and detoxifying

Examples: Fenugreek, neem leaves

Benefit: Reduces inflammation in the body

The Ayurveda perspective: In cases of excess fluids and toxin accumulation in the body tissues, a dry food habit has to be followed to reduce it. Dry-property food is bitter in its taste and acts as a detoxifier because of its natural qualities. It helps the body get rid of excess water and clears the toxins from the channels.

For a kapha dominant, it is good to start the day with food rich in the air and ether elements to detoxify the system and eliminate excess fluids that have accumulated on the cellular level. A toxin-free system gives optimal circulation of the blood and a smooth function of the lymph drainage system.

2. Weight-Reducing

Properties: Astringent, light, and anti-inflammatory

Examples: Tea leaves, raw apple, pomegranate

Benefits: Reduces the water and fat content in the tissues

The Ayurveda perspective: A major part of our body is water, which protects our organs from dehydration and oxidization. But an excess of water and fat can create mucus (kapham) and congestion in the system and overall heaviness in the body. Compared to the other two forces, kapha holds the highest level of water and stores the greatest amount of fat in the body, which gives the skin extra moisture and anti-aging effects. But in the long run, the excess water can create health issues, especially in the lungs and throat. The anti-inflammatory effects of food and drink rich in the air and ether elements can reduce the water and fat content in the tissues, which helps to decrease body mass. Ayurveda recommends light food to reduce excess body weight, especially in situations where the accumulated fat is threatening the cardiac functions or the heaviness of the body is causing bone-related problems.

3. Healing

Properties: Bitter, astringent, and cooling

Example: Aloe vera

Benefit: Heals skin problems such as eczema and psoriasis

The Ayurveda perspective: For centuries, Ayurveda has treated hyper pitta symptoms with the healing properties of the air and ether elements. For example, skin problems such as psoriasis and eczema can be treated with the medicinal content of aloe vera by using the pulp of this curative plant externally on the infected area and internally by drinking its juice. Drinking aloe vera juice on an empty stomach in the morning can also cure symptoms such as ulcers or hyperacidity in the esophagus, stomach, and intestines when the right food structure and lifestyle are maintained according to the presently dominating elements.

FOOD GUIDELINES FOR
YOUR DOMINANT FORCE

According to Ayurveda, not only WHAT we eat but also WHEN we eat and HOW MUCH we eat matter in our quest to attain perfect health. That is why in this chapter I have put together the most important guidelines to follow according to which force you want to stabilize at present. For instance, if your dominating force is kapha, you would follow the guidelines to control the earth and water elements, and so forth.

· · · · · · · · · · · · ·

Though snacks are included in the daily diet in the following recommendations for all three forces, they should be consumed according to the function of your present digestive system. For example, if you have poor digestion at the moment, you can skip the snacks in between breakfast and lunch and between lunch and dinner to give your stomach enough time to digest the large meals. If you have good digestion at present, the recommended snacks will kindle the agni (the digestive fire) and help you maintain your metabolism, promoting good health and immunity.

Kapha-Pacifying Food Guidelines

There is no better health care for kapha than discipline in the diet. To maintain maximum immunity and health, kapha dominants need to wake up early, around 6:00 a.m., and drink a glass of lukewarm water mixed with ginger or cleansing herbs. This practice reduces the excess mucosa that often accumulates at the back of the tongue and inside the walls of the esophagus in a kapha-dominated body. At about 8:00 a.m., after a morning walk or exercise, drink a cup of plain black tea (without sugar or milk) as an aid to eliminate puffiness in the body, since tea leaves have anti-inflammatory properties that can absorb excess water in the tissues.

Just as a sponge absorbs water, a kapha-dominated body holds more liquid in the tissues than the other two dominants do, and if we don't squeeze it out in time with the help of proper exercise and anti-inflammatory food and drink, it can cause health problems in the long run.

One of the most challenging practices for kapha dominants is to avoid eating before 10:00 a.m., considering that the period between 4:00 a.m. and 10:00 a.m. is the strongest kapha-influencing time in nature. If you are a kapha dominant, whatever you eat during these early hours of the day can create more ama (toxins), which accumulates in the body and increases body mass and decreases immune power. If you are striving to lose excess weight and improve your immunity, you can wait to eat breakfast until 10:00 a.m. (only if you are a kapha dominant), and drink warm water or tea during those hours to dissolve your hunger .

Every time you are in front of your food, remind yourself that you are eating to live, not living to eat. This mindset makes all the difference in your eating habits and encourages you, as a kapha dominant, to eat a light breakfast and dinner and make lunch your main meal of the day. Regardless of the season, as long as kapha is your PDE, make sure you do not eat before 10:00 a.m. or after 6:00 p.m. If you feel extremely hungry outside of your recommended eating hours, I suggest that you eat a piece of fruit such as an apple or drink some herbal tea or warm water.

To get a clear picture of the characteristics of the types of food that can reduce kapha, keep in mind that food that tastes bitter, astringent, or pungent is the best option. At the same time, food that is heavy, cold, or oily in its character and food that tastes sweet, salty, or sour are not good for kapha dominants and have to be avoided, since they can aggravate the force of kapha by causing an imbalance in the earth and water elements. I have noticed that plant-based food cooked with the right spices works well with the kapha metabolism, since most vegetables have the properties of bitter and astringent and the spices are pungent. So for a kapha dominant, there is nothing better to maintain the vitality than having a plant-based meal prepared with the right amount of spices.

Among my kapha dominant clients, I have noticed that the ones who reduce the quantity of their food intake and increase the quality of their diet by keeping a daily food diary and following a regular time-table for eating and drinking experience the best results from their food therapy, together with the disciplines of drinking less, avoiding drinking while eating, and staying away from cold beverages. Let's take a look at a healthy diet plan for a kapha dominant from the Ayurveda perspective.

Breakfast

Time: 10:00 a.m.

Quantity/Quality: Small and light

Recommendations: Light, dry food

Sample: Hard rye bread with a thin layer of herb paste and a bed of greens or sprouts, or a green smoothie or juice

Note: Morning (from 4:00 a.m. to 10:00 a.m.) is the most kapha-aggravating time, and kapha dominants need to refrain from doing anything that can increase the force of kapha. One of the best disciplines to balance kapha is to wake up early and eat as late as possible in the morning, or at least try to avoid eating breakfast during the early hours of kapha (4:00 a.m. to 8:00 a.m.) and avoid sleeping after 7:00 a.m.

Remember: If you have excess weight and are planning to reduce your body mass, you can skip breakfast and eat lunch as the first meal of the day.

Lunch

Time: Around 12:30 p.m.

Quantity/Quality: Light and warm

Recommendations: Protein-rich food with low levels of carbohydrates, and as fat-free as possible

Sample: Quinoa with vegetable or bean curry prepared with spices

Note: To keep the kapha force under control, lunch should be the only big meal of the day.

Remember: Stop drinking at least half an hour before a meal. This supports the agni, which we need to digest food properly. Kapha dominants have a tendency toward slow digestion, and for this reason they should avoid drinking during meals, thirty minutes before a meal, and two hours after a meal.

Tea Break

Time: 3:30 p.m.

Quantity/Quality: Small and light

Recommendations: Try to focus on your tea and eat the biscuits only if you really need to.

Sample: Biscuits or crackers without sugar or fat, with a cup of herbal kapha-balancing tea, such as clove or star anise or cinnamon tea. (To prepare this kapha-balancing tea, boil one of these spices in water for five minutes on low heat.) An apple or pomegranates also make a good kapha snack.

Note: If you are packing your snack, bring only one or two biscuits and avoid putting the full package in your snack box.

Remember: Apart from the tea break, don't eat anything between lunch and dinner, since your stomach needs enough time to digest the meal you had at lunch.

Dinner

Time: Between 5:30 and 6:00 p.m.

Quantity/Quality: Small

Recommendations: Make sure your dinner is warm and doesn't make you feel heavy.

Sample: Soup, such as spinach or ginger beetroot soup

Note: Eating an early dinner is one of the healthiest routines for kapha dominants. For the digestive system of a kapha type, the best time to eat dinner is before or at 6:00 p.m. Eating in the late evening creates ama (toxins) in the system and leads to problems such as fatigue and obesity.

Remember: Try to avoid eating after dinner. If you feel hunger or thirst, eat an apple or drink herbal tea before sleep.

Food and Mind Correlation for Kapha Dominants

Kapha dominants have to remember not to see food as a way to fill the empty spaces in their mind. From my experience with kapha-dominated clients, I have seen that they have a tendency during various periods of their life to have an emotional attachment to their food, which is one of the dangerous habits for this type, since they can easily fall in love with food, especially unhealthy foods and beverages. Though sweet is kapha-aggravating, they often get caught in an addiction to this taste, which makes it harder for them to get back into healthy habits. Because of the uncontrolled eating habits, once they become overweight, they may develop a self-pitying attitude and find excuses to treat themselves to more of the wrong foods and end up in a state of depression and misery in their life.

If you are a kapha dominant, try to avoid eating when you are sad or depressed, because it not only creates heaviness in the body but also causes difficulties in the normal function of the mind, such as a bad memory and a lack of clarity and sharpness in the brain function. This can manifest as extremely slow speech or difficulty making decisions and acting on them. To combat these health issues, my recommendation for all kapha dominants is to eat a light and disciplined diet and to see food merely as fuel for the body, not a way to fill your mind.

Food Recommendations for Kapha Dominants

Use the food chart in chapter 11 to learn which food items reduce or increase kapha. If your prakruti is kapha, your focus should be on adding the items in the "Kapha Favor" list to your diet and gradually reducing the items in the "Kapha Avoid/Reduce" list. If you have a kapha vikruti at the moment, strictly avoid the items in the "Kapha Avoid/Reduce" list and use only the items in the "Kapha Favor" list.

Pitta-Pacifying Food Guidelines

Considering the strength of the agni (fire) in this force, if pitta dominants are eating regularly, at the correct times, and in sufficient portions, then their intense and efficient digestive system is a gift; but if not, it can be a curse. As we learned earlier, pitta dominants have a powerful digestion and metabolism and need to eat regularly for a smooth function of the digestive system. If you, as a pitta dominant, fail to feed yourself on time, you are at risk of experiencing the symptoms of a fire and water imbalance, which starts with hyperacidity or a blistering sensation in the stomach. If your body is dominated by the force of pitta, drink a glass of water when you wake up and eat breakfast no later than 8:00 a.m., plus a morning snack around 10:00 a.m. as a filler between your breakfast and lunch.

Pitta dominants are sensitive and often overreact to many factors internally and externally, but I have noticed that their main struggles are excess heat and hunger. Through the right food planning, pitta dominants can regulate their body's heating system, as well as their appetite, with cooling-property foods and drinks. During the day, drink plenty of pure water to regulate the internal heat and hydrate the system. While I recommend that you drink enough, keep in mind that that doesn't mean to drink any beverage, such as caffeinated drinks or artificially flavored sodas, which will only dehydrate you and increase your thirst and heat instead of calming your system.

I have learned from my pitta dominant clients that they sometimes, or even for longer periods in their busy lives, forget to eat according to the signals from their stomach, which they end up paying for in the form of health disorders later on. Pitta dominants who neglect their hunger pangs risk turning their acidity into ulcers and tumors in the long run, causing immense pain and discomfort in the stomach. Always keep to your mealtimes, and don't let anything delay your regular eating times for any reason. It is not worth inviting problems into your body by compromising the most enjoyable moments in your life—your mealtimes—and then later trying to fix your issues with pills and surgeries.

When you wake up in the morning, in addition to your usual planning of what to do that day, make a quick plan in your mind about your natural medicine for the day: your food. For instance, if you are going out for a few hours, make sure you have some idea of where you are going to eat your meals during the day. Bring some fruit or natural snack bars with you as an emergency solution. Every time you feel your stomach churning with the call of hunger, eat a snack or, if it's your usual mealtime, take a break from your current activities and have your meal on time.

To get a general idea of the characteristics of food that can pacify pitta, consult the list of foods in the "Pitta Favor" section of the chart in chapter 11, which taste sweet, bitter, and astringent. But don't be too happy about my recommendation to add "sweet" to your food; when I say *sweet*, I mean natural foods with that property, such as grains and fruits, not processed sweets like chocolate or ice cream, made with the concentrated form of refined sugar. Ayurveda considers sugar to be white poison, and the use of it can put the health of your internal organs at risk. So make sure you choose your sweets wisely. Also avoid or reduce the use of salty, sour, and spicy foods in your daily diet, which can aggravate pitta and show up as symptoms in the body.

Studying the health of my pitta-dominated clients, I can say that even though they are sensitive to many external factors and prone to get colds and flu, if they are taking good care of their health with the recommended food lists of Ayurveda, they can maintain good health in any climate and at any age of their life. Let's take a look at a healthy food plan for a pitta dominant through the window of Ayurveda.

Breakfast

Time: Around 7:00 a.m.

Quantity/Quality: Wholesome

Recommendations: Grains, fresh vegetables, seeds, dried fruit

Sample: Dark bread with salad or sprouts and hummus (without garlic), porridge or a farmer's breakfast

Note: Pitta dominants need a quality breakfast because of the high digestive fire (agni) in their system.

Remember: When you eat your breakfast, be sure to sit down and allow enough time to enjoy your food.

Snack

Time: Around 10:00 a.m.

Quantity/Quality: Sweet

Recommendations: Fruit, seeds, or dried fruit (preferably dates)

Sample: A fresh smoothie made of fruits, or dry fruits and seeds, or biscuits made from healthy ingredients

Note: Pitta dominants can suffer from low blood pressure because of the hot nature of their system. A suitable snack can help regulate this.

Remember: Pack a snack if you are going to be out.

Lunch

Time: Around 12:30 p.m.

Quantity/Quality: Big and rich (largest meal of the day)

Recommendations: Carbohydrates prepared in less oil and with minimal spices

Sample: Amaranth, basmati rice, or couscous with steam-cooked or less-fried vegetables. Some recommended beans can be added in small amounts.

Note: Find enough time for your lunch. Before you eat, sit for at least seven seconds in silence and gently take three long breaths. This action gives you time to awaken your senses and redirect your focus to your food, which helps you enjoy it the most. Forget about everything else around you when you start eating your meal. Through these practices, you are upgrading and transforming your mealtime into a meditation, which is one of the daily meditation practices I suggest for your mind development and to live more in the moment.

Remember: Try to avoid fast and processed foods. Each time you eat an easy and fast lunch, remember that you are missing out on an opportunity to nourish your body with nature's real essence.

Tea Break

Time: Around 3:30 p.m.

Quantity/Quality: Cooling, grounding

Recommendations: Herbal tea, grains, fruits, vegetables

Sample: Tea made from pitta-balancing herbs or spices; healthy pitta-balancing bread with a spread made of plant-based ingredients

Note: Potato or sweet potato bread, as well as bread made with seeds and coconut, is pitta-balancing.

Remember: Try to avoid spicy teas.

Dinner

Time: Around 6:30 p.m.

Quantity/Quality: Second biggest meal of the day

Recommendations: Vegetables, grains, beans

Sample: Potato curry or vegetable stew, or a vegetable korma

Note: A mild curry with a coconut base is the perfect dish to stabilize pitta.

Remember: In a pitta-balancing dish, mild spices and herbs can be added, such as turmeric, dill, or mint.

Food and Mind Correlation for Pitta Dominants

To enjoy your food even after you have eaten and to make it your natural medicine, prepare your food with ingredients that come directly from nature, and always try to eat in a peaceful environment. Remember, your food is not just something to fill your stomach with, but is meant to fill your body and mind with nourishment and satisfaction. That is why I suggest that you do not eat when you are angry or irritated. In those situations, try to sit down with closed eyes and take a few deep, slow breaths until your mind is calm and ready to enjoy your food with complete focus.

If you are a pitta dominant, avoid nonvegetarian food, since it holds rajasic guna (excess fire), which can kindle negative emotions in your mind. Considering the fact that food is our vital energy source, and the healthiest sources of food are the ones we receive directly from nature, all the indirect sources of food that we ingest through the carcasses of animals lead to high levels of ama (toxins) in our system, and can cause several types of life-threatening diseases in the long run. From now on, let's make a promise to ourselves not to make our food plate a funeral place for dead animals.

Food Recommendations for Pitta Dominants

Use the food chart in chapter 11 to learn which food items reduce or increase pitta. If your prakruti is pitta, your focus should be on adding the items in the "Pitta Favor" list to your diet and reducing the items in the "Pitta Avoid/Reduce" list. If you have a pitta vikruti at the moment, strictly avoid the items in the "Pitta Avoid/Reduce" list and use only the items in the "Pitta Favor" list.

Vata-Pacifying Food Guidelines

For a vata dominant, the major challenge when it comes to food is discipline. As we know, our food won't just magically appear out of thin air and land on our plate when we want to eat. We need to plan and prepare before we can have our meal, and since vata dominants are poor planners in general, many times it becomes difficult for them to treat themselves with the right foods for their dominating elements. For this reason, I will provide a few steps here that are easier to follow, even for a person who normally doesn't follow any kind of discipline.

Start your morning with a glass of warm water. In between sips of water, place the warm glass on your chest and stomach and move it from left to right to warm yourself. Enhance your breakfast by adding digestion-supporting ingredients such as plant-based yogurt, grapes, or sour fruits. The vata digestive system has an irregular function, and this will generate hunger for the coming hours.

Vata dominants often have joint pain and itchy skin due to a lack of lubrication in the joints and extra dryness in the skin. This problem can be solved by eating a diet based on food that has oily and moisturizing characteristics. For instance, if you are suffering from extra dryness in the skin, eyes (sclera), mouth, the inner walls of the nostrils, or the anal cavities, or are feeling pain in the joints, you can add oily food to your diet. For example, add avocado to your diet and treat your health issues with the support of Mother Nature.

Food and lifestyle are very important factors when balancing the forces, and since a good night's sleep is essential to the function of the digestive system of vata dominants, considering their sensitivity to sleep, they need to take special care in all three of these areas to maintain better health and immunity. Since everything is interrelated, food and sleep can complement each other. So eating a grounding dinner, like warm soup with the right amount of spices, can help the air and ether elements stay balanced in the system and promote a good digestion and a sound sleep during the night.

The best thing about being a vata dominant is that, compared to the other two dominants, you can eat most of the food items in nature if you know how to maintain your agni, the digestive fire in your system. As a vata dominant, if your digestion is not powerful enough at the moment, you can eat small portions of food mixed with digestion-aiding spices. And once you regain your digestive fire, you can maintain it by eating the same amount of food at the same time every day. Though this can be a hard discipline for vata dominants, from my experience with my clients, the ones who follow the Ayurveda recommendations with the proper discipline get the best results not only in their digestion and metabolism but also in the quality of their sleep.

To get a clear picture in your mind of vata-balancing food, think of the foods that taste sweet, salty, and sour, then find these items from natural sources and implement them in your diet. At the same time, try to avoid food that has an astringent taste and reduce the use of the pungent and bitter tastes. Since most vegetables taste bitter and astringent, and spices are naturally pungent, I can understand how you might feel while reading these words if you are a vata dominant and a veggie lover. Well, like my grandma often reminded me, there is always a solution to every problem, and in this case that is absolutely true. This means that even though most vegetables have vata-increasing properties in their natural state, when you cook them properly and mix them with the right spices, their natural properties dissolve and won't be of any harm, as would be the case if you ate them in their raw form. So try to find good recipes to prepare your veggies. If you want to look into some dishes from my village, you can find them on my website.

Though all dominations have advantages in some areas and disadvantages in others, vata dominants are the most fortunate when it comes to food, since they have much more freedom than the other two dominants to choose their food. The only thing they need to make sure of is to constantly kindle their minimum digestive fire with the right spices to maintain their digestion and immune power.

Breakfast

Time: Around 8:00 to 8:30 a.m.

Quantity/Quality: Warm and grounding

Recommendations: Cooked grains, spices, fruit

Sample: Ayurveda farmer's breakfast or oatmeal porridge with spices and banana or cooked apples

Note: Vata dominants need food with warm and nourishing properties right at the beginning of the day to feel grounded.

Remember: Stay away from cold smoothies and juices in the morning.

Snack

Time: Around 10:00 to 10:30 a.m.

Quantity/Quality: Warm with spices

Recommendations: Herbal spice tea

Sample: Tea made from vata-balancing spices, with a snack such as soft ginger or sesame cookies

Note: If the temperature outside is warm, you can exchange your morning snack for one of the suggestions for your afternoon tea break.

Remember: Use discipline and plan ahead so you always have a snack handy at the right time.

Lunch

Time: Around 12:30 p.m.

Quantity/Quality: Warm and nourishing

Recommendations: Carbohydrates and protein-rich combinations cooked in enough oil and spices

Sample: Steam-cooked vegetables such as carrots, sweet potatoes, or yams, plus grain combinations such as rice cooked with bits of almonds, or beans prepared in hot spices

Note: According to a person's culture and the climate, the preparation methods and flavors of the food can vary from country to country.

Remember: Focus on your food as you prepare and eat it. Chew your food properly and pay attention to your breathing while eating.

Tea Break

Time: Around 3:30 p.m.

Quantity/Quality: Sweet

Recommendation: Fruit at room temperature

Sample: Vata-balancing fruit such as mango, orange, grapes, or papaya at room temperature, as juice, or in raw form

Note: Be creative with your fruit: cut it in interesting shapes, make a fruit skewer, etc.

Remember: Do not eat frozen fruit or fruit straight from the refrigerator.

Dinner

Time: Around 6:30 p.m.

Quantity/Quality: Warm and grounding

Recommendations: Grains and cooked vegetables

Sample: Couscous and vegetables cooked with a sauce and spices

Note: All black beans are highly vata-increasing and should be avoided for dinner. Mung beans or red lentils are fine to eat as a soup if prepared with enough spices and cooked onions.

Remember: You can make your own combinations, but remember not to combine two heavy food items—for instance, grains and beans or nightshade foods and beans—which can cause indigestion in the stomach for vata dominants, especially in the evening.

Food and Mind Correlation for Vata Dominants

Considering that food is the life-saving fuel of the body, if you are a vata dominant, take extra care in all areas of your diet, from shopping to cooking to eating. Avoid eating when you feel anxious, worried, or stressed, since the body will be focused on the release of adrenaline and other stress-related hormones such as cortisol, and your digestive system won't function optimally. As a result, the undigested food will generate ama (toxins) in the system and obstruct the natural functions of your immune cells.

In such situations of uneasiness in the mind, try to sit with closed eyes and say a silent prayer in front of your food, contemplating your thoughts about the food you are about to celebrate. Silently give thanks to the farmer who cultivated your food and to Mother Nature, who fed the crops with rain, dried it with the sun, and combed it with the wind. Be imaginative and look at your food with loving eyes. Be patient with each molecule of food you place inside your mouth, and chew it several times, feeling the joy of melting nature's healing essences on your taste buds while making love to the flavors on the bed of your tongue, feeling satisfaction and joy with every bite of your food.

Food Recommendations for Vata Dominants

Use the food chart in chapter 11 to learn which food items reduce or increase vata. If your prakruti is vata, your focus should be on adding the items in the "Vata Favor" list to your diet and reducing the items in the "Vata Avoid/Reduce" list. If you have a vata vikruti at the moment, you should avoid the items in the "Vata Avoid/Reduce" list and use only the items from the "Vata Favor" list.

FOOD CHART TO BALANCE
THE ELEMENTS IN YOUR SYSTEM

The food chart in this chapter is based on the traditional knowledge of Ayurveda that I received from my ancestors in India, as well as my research of nature's healing foods for over fifteen years in Europe and the United States. This chart is for people in search of the healthiest food sources from nature to promote optimal health and immune power.

·············

While plant-based food is the primary source of our energy, all other forms of food, such as the food that comes from animals and their byproducts, is a secondary source of food, since we are then receiving the plant energy through an animal body that once received the energy from plants. While eating a plant-based diet makes our stomach function better and keeps our mind calm, an animal-based diet boosts the stress levels in our mind and leaves ama (toxins) in our system, making our organs prone to infectious and noninfectious diseases.

In the following chart, you will find the sources of food that are recommended to balance your presently dominating elements and thus maintain optimal good health and immunity. I have prepared this food chart with consideration of the practicality of your food shopping and cooking in mind. In the chart you can find the vegetables, legumes, grains, nuts and seeds, oils, and spices that you need to add to your diet to balance your presently dominating elements. (For a regularly updated version of this food chart, visit the Ayurveda food section of my website at janeshvaidya.com/ayurveda/food/.)

It is good to keep in mind that there are some food items whose natural qualities can change during the cooking process. That means that even though some food ingredients are not good for your PDE (presently dominating elements), with the right cooking techniques and combination of spices, you can use those ingredients in moderation, which I have indicated in the chart with star combinations. While a single star (*) after an item means to use that item only in moderation, double stars (**) after an item indicate to use that item only when properly cooked. You will also see items marked with three stars and a space in between (* **), which means that you should use that item only in moderation and only when it is properly cooked.

Kapha Avoid/Reduce	
Vegetables	**Fruit**
Ash gourd*	Avocado
Bottle gourd	Banana
Cassava	Blackberries*
Cucumber	Blueberries*
Olives (green and black)	Coconut
Parsnip*	Dates
Pumpkin	Figs (fresh)
Ridge gourd	Grapefruit
Squash	Green grapes
Sweet potato	Kiwi
Taro root	Melon
Tomato (cooked)*	Orange
Tomato (raw)	Papaya
Yam	Pineapple
Zucchini	Plums
	Rhubarb
	Tamarind
	Watermelon
Grains	**Legumes**
Couscous*	Chickpeas*
Durum flour*	Kidney beans*
Oats (cooked)	
Rice (white)	
Spelt*	
Wheat	
*Use only in moderation ** Use only when properly cooked*	
*** Use only in moderation and only when properly cooked*	

Kapha Avoid/Reduce (*continued*)	
Nuts & Seeds	**Oil**
Almond (soaked and peeled)*	Almond oil*
Brazil nut	Apricot oil
Cashew	Avocado oil
Hazelnut	Coconut oil
Hempseed	Olive oil
Macadamia nut	Primrose oil
Peanut	Sesame oil
Pecan	Soybean oil
Pine nut	Walnut oil
Pistachios	**Spices & Herbs**
Sesame seed	Salt*
Walnut	Vanilla*

Kapha Favor	
Vegetables	**Fruit**
Artichoke*	Apple
Arugula	Apricot
Asparagus	Black/red/purple grapes*
Aubergine	Berries
Beetroot**	Cherries*
Bell pepper	Cranberries
Bitter melon	Figs (dry)*
Bok choy	Guava*
Broccoli	Lemon*
Brussels sprouts	Lime*
Burdock root	Lingonberries
Cabbage	Mango*
Carrot**	Peach*
Cauliflower	Pear
Celery	Persimmon
Chard	Pomegranate
Chayote squash	Prunes
* *Use only in moderation* ** *Use only when properly cooked*	
* ** *Use only in moderation and only when properly cooked*	

Kapha Favor (*continued*)	
Vegetables	**Fruit**
Chili	Raisins
Chinese potato	Raspberries*
Corn**	Strawberries*
Daikon radish	**Grains**
Dandelion greens	Amaranth
Drumstick leaves	Barley
Elephant foot yam**	Buckwheat
Fennel	Corn
Horseradish	Millet
Ivy gourd	Oats (dry)
Jerusalem artichoke	Polenta
Kale	Quinoa
Kohlrabi	Rice (basmati)*
Leafy greens	Rice (black)
Leek	Rice (brown)*
Lettuce	Rye
Mushroom*	Wild rice
Mustard greens	**Legumes**
Okra**	Adzuki beans
Onion	Black beans
Potato	Black-eyed peas
Radish	Green beans
Rutabaga	Lentils
Snake gourd	Lima beans
Spinach	Mung beans*
Sprouts	Mung beans (split)*
Sundried tomato*	Navy beans
Turnip	Peas (green)
Watercress	Peas (yellow)
	Pigeon peas (split)
	Pinto beans
	Soybeans*
	White beans

Kapha Favor (*continued*)	
Nuts & Seeds	**Oil**
Chia seeds	Canola oil*
Corn (popped without salt)	Corn oil*
Flaxseed*	Flaxseed oil*
Psyllium*	Mustard oil*
Pumpkin seed*	Safflower oil*
Sunflower seed*	Sunflower oil*

Spices & Herbs	
Ajwain	Fenugreek
Allspice	Garlic
Anise	Ginger
Asafetida	Long pepper
Basil	Mace
Bay leaf	Marjoram
Black pepper	Mint
Caraway	Mustard seed
Cardamom	Neem leaf
Cayenne	Nutmeg
Chili powder	Oregano
Cilantro	Paprika powder
Cinnamon	Parsley
Clove	Rosemary
Coriander powder	Saffron
Cumin	Sage
Curry leaves	Star anise
Dill	Tarragon
Fennel*	Thyme
	Turmeric

* Use only in moderation   ** Use only when properly cooked
* ** Use only in moderation and only when properly cooked

Pitta Avoid/Reduce	
Vegetables	**Fruit**
Aubergine*	Apples (sour)
Beetroot (cooked)*	Apricot (sour)
Beetroot (raw)	Banana*
Burdock root	Berries (sour)
Carrot (cooked)*	Cherries (sour)
Carrot (raw)	Cranberries
Chard	Grapefruit
Chili	Green grapes (sour)
Corn (fresh)*	Kiwi*
Daikon radish	Lemon*
Drumstick leaves	Lingonberries*
Elephant foot yam	Mango (less ripe)
Horseradish	Orange (sour)
Kohlrabi*	Papaya*
Leek (raw)	Peach
Mustard greens	Persimmon
Olive (green)	Pineapple (less ripe)
Onion (cooked)*	Plum (sour)
Onion (raw)	Raspberries*
Pumpkin*	Rhubarb
Radish	Tamarind (sour)
Spinach (cooked)*	**Legumes**
Spinach (raw)	Lentils*
Sprouts (pungent)	Pigeon peas (split)
Sundried tomato	
Tomato	
Turnip	
Watercress*	
Yam*	

Pitta Avoid/Reduce (*continued*)	
Grains	**Nuts & Seeds**
Buckwheat	Almond
Corn	Brazil nut
Millet	Cashew
Oats (dry)	Chia seeds*
Polenta*	Hazelnut
Rice (brown)*	Macadamia
Rye	Peanut
Spices & Herbs	Pecan
Ajwain	Pine nut
Allspice	Pistachios
Anise	Sesame seed
Asafetida	Walnut
Basil (dry)	**Oil**
Bay leaf	Apricot oil
Black pepper*	Corn oil
Cayenne	Flaxseed oil*
Curry leaves*	Mustard oil
Fenugreek	Olive oil*
Garlic	Peanut oil
Ginger (dry)	Safflower oil
Long pepper	Sesame oil
Mace	
Marjoram	* *Use only in moderation*
Mustard seeds	** *Use only when properly cooked*
Nutmeg	* ** *Use only in moderation and*
Oregano	*only when properly cooked*
Paprika	
Paprika powder	
Rosemary*	
Sage	
Salt*	
Star anise	
Thyme	

Pitta Favor	
Vegetables	**Fruit**
Artichoke	Apple (sweet)
Arugula	Apricots (sweet)
Ash gourd	Avocado*
Asparagus	Berries (sweet)
Bell pepper	Blackberries (ripe)*
Bitter melon	Black/red/purple grapes (sweet)
Bok choy	Blueberries (ripe)
Bottle gourd	Cherries (sweet)
Broccoli	Coconut
Brussels sprouts	Dates
Cabbage	Figs
Cassava	Guava
Cauliflower	Lime*
Celery	Mango (ripe)
Chayote squash*	Melon
Chinese potato*	Orange (sweet)*
Cucumber	Pear
Dandelion greens	Pineapple (ripe)
Fennel	Plums (sweet)
Ivy gourd	Pomegranate
Jerusalem artichoke	Prunes
Kale	Raisins
Leafy greens (mild)	Strawberries*
Leek (cooked)	Watermelon

* *Use only in moderation*   ** *Use only when properly cooked*
* ** *Use only in moderation and only when properly cooked*

Pitta Favor (*continued*)	
Vegetables (*continued*)	**Grains**
Lettuce	Amaranth
Mushroom*	Barley
Okra	Couscous
Olives (black)	Durum flour
Parsnip	Oats (cooked)
Potato	Quinoa*
Ridge gourd	Rice (basmati)
Rutabaga*	Rice (white)
Snake gourd	Spelt
Sprouts (mild)	Wheat*
Squash	**Nuts & Seeds**
Sweet potato	Almond (soaked and peeled)*
Taro root	Corn (popped without salt)
Zucchini	Flaxseed
Legumes	Hempseed*
Adzuki beans*	Psyllium
Black beans	Pumpkin seed*
Black-eyed peas	Sunflower seed
Chickpeas	**Oil**
Green beans	Almond oil*
Kidney beans	Avocado oil*
Lima beans*	Canola oil
Mung beans	Coconut oil
Mung beans (split)	Primrose oil
Navy beans	Soybean oil
Peas	Sunflower oil
Pinto beans	Walnut oil*
Soybeans	
White beans	
* *Use only in moderation* ** *Use only when properly cooked*	
* ** *Use only in moderation and only when properly cooked*	

Pitta Favor (*continued*)	
Spices & Herbs	
Basil (fresh)*	Fennel
Caraway*	Ginger (fresh)*
Cardamom*	Mint
Cilantro	Neem leaf*
Cinnamon*	Parsley
Clove*	Saffron*
Coriander powder	Tarragon*
Cumin	Turmeric
Dill	Vanilla*

Vata Avoid/Reduce		
Vegetables	**Fruit**	
Artichoke*	Apple	
Arugula*	Banana (unripe)	
Aubergine	Cranberries	
Bell pepper**	Dates (dry)	
Bitter melon	Figs (dry)	
Broccoli	Guava	
Brussels sprouts	Lingonberries	
Burdock root	Pear	
Cabbage (raw)	Persimmon	
Cauliflower (cooked)* **	Pomegranate	
Cauliflower (raw)	Prunes (dry)	
Celery	Raisins (dry)	
Chard*	Watermelon	
Chayote squash	**Grains**	
Chinese potato* **	Barley	Polenta*
Corn (fresh)	Buckwheat*	Quinoa (puffed)
Dandelion greens	Corn*	Rye
Ivy gourd*	Millet	Spelt
Jerusalem artichoke*	Oats (dry)	
Kale		

Vata Avoid/Reduce (*continued*)	
Vegetables (*continued*)	**Legumes**
Kohlrabi	Adzuki beans* **
Leafy greens*	Black beans* **
Lettuce*	Black-eyed peas* **
Mushroom	Broad beans
Olive (green)*	Chickpeas* **
Onion (raw)	Kidney beans* **
Potato	Lentils (brown/green)
Radish (raw)	Lima beans
Ridge gourd	Navy beans
Snake gourd*	Peas (dried)
Spinach (raw)	Peas (raw)
Squash (raw)	Pinto beans* **
Sundried tomato*	Soybeans* **
Tomato (cooked)*	White beans
Tomato (raw)	**Nuts & Seeds**
Turnip	Corn (popped)
Zucchini (raw)	
Oil	**Spices & Herbs**
Canola oil*	Cayenne pepper*
Corn oil*	Chili powder*
Soybean oil*	Fenugreek*
	Neem leaves*
* *Use only in moderation* ** *Use only when properly cooked*	
* ** *Use only in moderation and only when properly cooked*	

Vata Favor	
Vegetables	**Fruit**
Ash gourd	Apples (cooked)
Asparagus	Apricot
Beetroot	Avocado
Bottle gourd	Banana
Cabbage (cooked)*	Berries
Carrot	Blackberries
Cassava* **	Blueberries
Chili*	Cherries
Corn (cooked)*	Coconut
Cucumber	Dates (fresh, soaked, or cooked)
Daikon radish*	Figs (fresh, soaked, or cooked)
Drumstick leaves	Grapefruit
Elephant foot yam	Grapes
Fennel	Kiwi
Horseradish*	Lemon
Leek	Lime
Okra	Mango
Olive (black)	Melon
Onion (cooked)*	Orange
Parsnip	Papaya
Pumpkin	Peach
Radish (cooked)*	Pineapple
Rutabaga**	Plums
Seaweed	Prunes (soaked or cooked)
Spinach (cooked)*	Raisins (soaked or cooked)
Sprouts*	Raspberries*
Squash (cooked)*	Rhubarb
Sweet potato	Strawberries
Taro root	Tamarind
Watercress	
Yam	
Zucchini (cooked)	

Vata Favor (*continued*)	
Grains	**Legumes**
Amaranth★	Green beans (cooked)
Couscous★	Lentils (red)
Durum flour	Mung beans
Oats (cooked)	Mung beans (split)
Quinoa (cooked)★	Peas (cooked)
Rice	Pigeon peas (split)
Wheat	Vegan paneer★
Nuts & Seeds	**Oil**
Almond	Almond oil
Brazil nut	Avocado oil
Cashew nut★	Coconut oil★
Chia seeds	Flaxseed oil★
Flaxseed	Mustard oil
Hazelnut	Olive oil
Hempseed	Peanut oil
Macadamia nut	Sesame oil
Peanut★	**Spices & Herbs**
Pecan nut	Ajwain
Pine nut	Allspice
Pistachios	Anise
Psyllium★	Asafetida
Pumpkin seed	Basil
Sesame seed	Bay leaf
Sunflower seeds	Black pepper
Walnut	Caraway
★ *Use only in moderation* ★★ *Use only when properly cooked* ★ ★★ *Use only in moderation and only when properly cooked*	

Vata Favor (*continued*)	
Spices & Herbs	
Cardamom	Mustard seed
Cilantro	Nutmeg
Cinnamon	Oregano
Clove	Paprika powder
Coriander powder*	Parsley
Cumin	Rosemary
Curry leaves	Saffron
Dill	Sage*
Fennel	Salt
Garlic*	Star anise
Ginger	Tarragon
Long pepper	Thyme
Mace	Turmeric
Marjoram	Vanilla
Mint	

Part 3
LIFESTYLE—
THE KEY TO YOUR HEALTH

There are two kind of factors that influence our health and immunity: direct and indirect factors. While global climate changes indirectly affect our life, threatening our health from a distance, other factors directly affect us, constantly disturbing our mind-body systems.

Even though the worsening climatic conditions around the world are not under our total individual control, it is good to remember that all the shifts from the original state of our planet's elements have an influence on the health and immunity of the living species on it. For instance, pollution of the air, water, and earth is increasing every day around the world, warming the ocean and melting the ice in the arctic regions. These polar ice caps are the refrigerator of our planet, and through decades of global warming caused by pollution, a major part of it has already melted, accelerating the climatic changes through the shifts of our planet's structural elements: earth, water, fire, air, and ether. These drastic changes in the ratio of the elements affect our ecosystem, threatening the health and existence of every species on this planet, including humans.

To control pollution and global warming, we need a collective effort from our society, which we need to see as a long-term project, even though we want to save our planet and preserve the constitutional elements of Mother Nature as soon as we can. If we all consider our part in generating pollution and attempt to reduce it in our daily lives by returning to an eco-friendly lifestyle, we can achieve this goal in the near future. However, saving the planet requires the cooperation of the people in our society. We need to open the eyes of the leaders in our country and raise the awareness of the entire world to the urgency of this essential change. So what can we do now?

Let's take a look at the factors directly influencing our health through the elements of our internal and external nature that form the forces and control our mind-body system throughout our life. While the birth- and age-dominating elements influence our body from the inside, the seasons and the time of day influence our system from the outside, and govern our health and immunity during our lifetime. As explained previously, we can't change our birth dominating elements that make up the qualities and limitations of our core personality. And we also can't control the natural aging process, the changing seasons in nature, and the passing of time during the day. So the question is, if we can't directly change any of these health-influencing factors in our life, how can we improve our health and our immune power?

Although we can't control the above factors influencing our health directly or indirectly with our personal choices, we can reduce their harmful effects. When we make conscious choices in our daily life, we can even reduce the effect of global climatic changes on our health and immunity to an extent.

Ayurveda teaches us the important lesson that by making the right lifestyle changes according to your prakruti or vikruti, you can control the effects of the external forces. You can eliminate the over-aging process and the worst impact of the imbalanced elements that aggravate the corresponding forces, generating symptoms and diseases in the body. In this third part of our studies, let us discuss what we can do in our own lives to improve our health and immunity with the right lifestyle changes.

IMMUNE-BOOSTING
LIFESTYLE HABITS

Before we proceed to the lifestyle recommendations for each domination,
let us get acquainted with the general habits that influence our health.
The first chart in this chapter gives us clues to which habits promote
health and which habits put our health at risk.

. . . .

We have learned that while a balanced state of the elements in our body maintains health, an imbalanced state aggravates the associated forces (kapha, pitta, and vata) and weakens our immunity. The wrong diet, an undisciplined lifestyle, or unhealthy thoughts can cause imbalances in the natural levels of the elements. That means that our health depends on what we eat, how we live, and the attitude we have toward life.

Let us take a look at the general lifestyle habits that influence our health. The first column of the following chart lists the recommendations to follow for optimal health, where the practitioner chooses the right food, lifestyle, and mind practice according to their PDE. The last two columns list less healthy food and lifestyle habits, which pose risks to your health to a minor and major degree and are the habits you need to change to achieve maximum health.

Healthy and Unhealthy Diet, Lifestyle, and Mind Habits

Practice	Habits That Promote Health (*Choose as per your birth dominant/imbalanced elements*)	Minor Unhealthy Habits (*Try to reduce/avoid as much as possible*)	Major Unhealthy Habits (*Avoid/change*)
1. Diet			
Food	(Primary source of food)* Vegetables, fruits, spices, herbs, nuts, seeds, grains, and legumes	(Secondary source of food)** White meat, small fish	(Secondary source of food)** Red meat, large fish
Drinks	Pure water, herbal teas, fresh juices, and smoothies	Carbonated water, soft drinks, coffee, mild alcohol	Strong alcohol
2. Lifestyle			
Sleep/ rest	7–8 hours a day	More than 10 hours a day	Less than 4 hours a day
Physical exercise	Exercise according to your PDE— daily practice	Exercise without considering your PDE	Exercise while ignoring symptoms/imbalanced state of elements in the body
Sex drive	Constant—tantric (not focused on the orgasm)	Quick—focused on the final result (orgasm)	Suppressed love—not at all interested in sex
Work	For peace	For making money and accumulating material possessions	For destruction of life, including nature and animals

Healthy and Unhealthy Diet, Lifestyle, and Mind Habits (continued)

Practice	Habits That Promote Health (*Choose as per your birth dominant/ imbalanced elements*)	Minor Unhealthy Habits (*Try to reduce/ avoid as much as possible*)	Major Unhealthy Habits (*Avoid/change*)
3. Mind	Focused, enthusiastic, satisfied, pleasant, and peaceful	Worried, stressed, fearful, or anxious	Holding anger/ hate, long-term sadness/depression

* *Primary source of food:* Adapting the right plant-based diet according to the PDE increases the vitality and life energy of a human and thus reduces the risk of harmful microorganisms invading the body and generating diseases in the system.

** *Secondary source of food:* When humans eat animals to get the nourishment that the animal once received from plants, it is considered an indirect source of nourishment. The animal-based food enters the human stomach with ama (toxins) and harmful microorganisms, threatening the immune system and disturbing the balance of the elements and thus our health.

Since we are focusing on optimal health, I advise you to use alternatives to animal products and byproducts in your Ayurveda diet. For example, honey and dairy products such as milk, yogurt, and ghee can be replaced with plant-based options available at the store. In my Ayurveda retreat in South India, my family practices traditional Ayurveda disciplines, following completely plant-based food and treatment programs for the best health results for the guests, and peace for other lives on this planet.

Traditional Morning Routines to Optimize Your Energy

As my grandma used to say, "The morning is the best time to start a good habit. When you choose good thoughts in the morning, it creates good feelings for the day. And when you create good feelings every day, your mind will be more positive all week. And when you make your weeks and months and years positive, your entire life will be a cycle of positive energy."

Understanding the importance of having a positive morning, I introduce here five traditional Ayurveda practices that I learned from my grandma. With these morning practices, you will start your day with healthy habits and thus live the coming days, weeks, months, years, and your entire life the best way you can.

The morning routines in the following chart have been practiced by Vaidyas (the traditional Ayurveda practitioners in India) through several generations. Regardless of their presently dominating elements, anyone can practice these five steps in the morning and experience a boost in mental and physical energy in three weeks' time.

In India, people say to wake up with the sun, which is around 6:00 to 7:00 a.m. all year round. But in countries farther away from the equator, we need to change that time frame and use logic instead, considering the difference in the sun's transit.

According to the ancient health practices of my village, the early morning sunrays can heal many illnesses in our system. The sunlight improves agni, the fire element, which controls the immune power in the body, and the morning sun rejuvenates the brain and supports the production of hormones such as serotonin and dopamine, which are essential for our mental function.

Five Traditional Morning Routines to Optimize Your Energy

Step	Disciplines	Physical Practice	Mental Practice
1	Clear your mind.	When your mind wakes from sleep in the morning, instead of rising, stay in your bed for a couple of minutes, lying in savasana* and breathing gently, with eyes closed.	Be grateful for being alive today. Cultivate affirmative thoughts and connect with your positive feelings, contemplating what you would love to do today to fulfill your heart's wishes.
2	Clean your mouth and your mind.	Brush your teeth and tongue and massage your gums with your index fingers. (If you are following a clean, plant-based diet and you brush your teeth with toothpaste in the evening, you only need to use warm water to clean your teeth in the morning.) If you have any kapha symptoms, such as mucus congestion in the throat, gargle with warm saline water.	Look in the mirror with a smile from your heart, seeing a reflection of your good sides. Plan how you can invest your positive energies in the coming hours of the day to find joy and peace in your life, and prepare to greet the people you meet with a smile.

* *Savasana* is the corpse pose in yoga.

Five Traditional Morning Routines to Optimize Your Energy (continued)

Step	Disciplines	Physical Practice	Mental Practice
3	Cleanse your esophagus, stomach, and mind.	Practice water therapy** or drink an herbal tea as prescribed for your PDE.	Sit in a comfortable position, with a focused mind leading to affirmative thoughts. Drink slowly, as if you are eating the water/tea.
4	Eliminate waste particles and toxins from your intestines, and release tension from your belly.	Make a habit of sitting on the toilet for a few minutes in the morning after drinking the water/herbal tea. This routine helps the brain program the excretory organs to eliminate waste matter from the intestines every morning, even for people who have difficulty emptying the bowels regularly.	While sitting on the toilet, try to connect your mind to the bottom of your abdomen by placing your palms over your belly. Inhale, filling the diaphragm until the belly expands to its maximum, then exhale, gently drawing the belly toward the spine.
5	Vitalize your body and mind.	Follow your daily morning exercise/yoga therapy program.***	When you are on the yoga mat, keep your complete focus inward and observe your body from head to toe while making a rhythmic flow of breath through your inhalations and exhalations.

** You can find instructions for water therapy on my website.

*** You can find yoga therapy programs for your PDE in chapter 18.

Designing Your Lifestyle According to Your PDE

With this section, I want to make sure that you are well aware of your choices when it comes to taking charge of your health, and the steps to advance from one level of your health practice to another. We will also emphasize the importance of knowing your PDE when designing your lifestyle.

Ayurveda is a lifestyle, a healthy style that upgrades all areas of a person's life with the right application of this ancient wisdom. Since the disciplines and habits in our daily life play a major role in our physical and mental development, let us focus on making necessary lifestyle changes in the coming days.

A healthy lifestyle is not just doing some general exercises or following a trendy diet. Instead, it is the practice of your natural health by understanding the PDE (presently dominating elements) in your mind-body system and following a tailor-made program to maintain the stability of your dominating forces (kapha, pitta, and vata) in different seasons and at different ages of your life. When you follow your daily routines according to your PDE, you will see steady progress in your inner and outer health.

When you have laid the foundation for your health by starting your mornings with the Ayurveda disciplines in the previous chart, you will be one step ahead on your health journey. Now we can discuss how you can improve the rest of the hours in your daily life by designing a lifestyle according to your presently dominating elements.

With the help of the self-tests in chapter 5, you can determine the presently dominating elements of your mind-body system, which we call your PDE. As discussed earlier, your PDE can indicate your *prakruti*, the birth dominating elements, or your *vikruti*, the dysfunction of the body and mind caused by the highest aggravated force in the system.

Let me remind you of the following factors:

1. If you have an aggravation in any of the three forces (kapha, pitta, or vata), that is your vikruti, caused by an imbalanced state of your PDE.

2. If you have vikruti in more than one force, as when two forces or even all three forces (kapha, pitta, and vata) are aggravated at the same time, then the force with the highest vikruti among them is indicated by your PDE.

3. If you don't have an imbalance in any element (which means your present body and mind systems are functioning with no symptoms or diseases) and you have no signs of dysfunction in any organ/system, then your PDE (presently dominating elements) indicates your prakruti.

While in the first two conditions your PDE indicates your *vikruti*, in the third condition your PDE indicates your *prakruti*. (That means that in the absence of an imbalance in your body and mind, your presently dominating elements show your prakruti, indicating the highest force in your system at your birth). In all three conditions, you need to focus on balancing your PDE to maintain your ultimate health. While in the first two conditions you will focus on balancing the imbalanced elements, in the third condition your focus will be to maintain the balance of your birth dominating elements and thus maintain your health and immunity with the right food and lifestyle disciplines.

The Three Levels of a Health Practice

We often see people make lifestyle changes without considering the status of their present health. Even though any lifestyle change can be considered the first level of a health practice, if we only follow the trendy advice from the health industry without considering the aftereffects, our practice won't last too long and won't give us the results we seek.

Whether you are following a new diet or a popular workout program, without enough research of its direct and indirect impact on your body and mind over a longer period of time, it can only be considered a general exercise program. On the other hand, when you follow an individual program with the right knowledge and with an awareness of its effects on your system, it becomes your therapy, which is the second level of your health practice. Through the disciplined practice of an individual health program, you automatically upgrade your life to the next level, where you develop not only your physical and mental sides but also the spiritual aspects of your life.

From now on, think about how you make your choices in life: merely as an exercise, as a therapy, or even for your spiritual development? For instance, the food choices we make show what level of a health practice we are on right now. If we fill our stomach according to our addicted senses, without considering our present state of health, we can consider it an exercise in survival. In this state we are eating to maintain our addictions, not our health. When we give priority to our health, we eat the food that is best for our system, and by making that conscious choice, eating becomes a therapy and our food becomes our natural medicine. Now imagine that we are choosing our food not only according to the health status of our body and mind but also for our soul, searching for food with clean energy, which is the highest level of a health practice, nourishing the spiritual aspects of our life.

Always be aware of your choices in life and make decisions according to what level of improvements you are searching for. During most periods of your life, you can consider your health to be a conscious choice. Remind yourself that you have many choices, even during the hard times when you feel stuck and lost on the path of your life journey.

DAILY ROUTINES TO IMPROVE YOUR IMMUNE POWER

In this chapter I will explain how you can adapt your daily routines to fit your PDE, your presently dominating elements. The recommendations here include the best time to wake up, plus daytime activities and evening disciplines to optimize your health and immunity. We will also discuss the most common obstacles you may face when establishing a new lifestyle regimen, depending on your dominating elements.

············

The very first stage of moving into a healthy lifestyle is to start a discipline in the most vital areas in our daily life, such as food, exercise, and sleep. When our body needs energy, first of all we need to find the right food to feed our systems. To digest the food and distribute it with ease to the tissues, we need to practice the right exercises. And when our internal systems have been working for a while, our body gets tired and requires rest in order for the systems to repair and refresh themselves through sufficient sleep. This is the healthy routine that needs to be repeated in a day-night cycle to maintain our natural immune power and thus attain a healthy body and mind. And if we can establish a routine for these three necessities (the right food, the right exercise, and enough rest) in our daily life, then we are one step closer to better health. In this chapter you will find traditional Ayurveda recommendations to design a routine according to your PDE (presently dominating elements), which controls the dominating force in your body and mind at the moment.

Daily Routines to Stabilize Kapha

Wake Up Early

The period from 4:00 a.m. to 10:00 a.m. is the most kapha-aggravating time of the day. People with kapha prakruti or vikruti need to wake up early to avoid the influence of the earth and water elements from nature during these hours. Kapha dominants should avoid sleeping in the late hours of the morning; otherwise there is a risk of water-related symptoms such as excess mucus causing sinusitis, heaviness in the head, and congestion in the throat and lungs.

Drink a Glass of Warm Water with Ginger

The root of *Zingiber officinale* (ginger) is an immune booster because of its ability to kindle the agni, the fire element in the system. With the support of ginger, agni can enhance the heat in the digestive and circulatory systems, reduce inflammation, and burn fat in the body. Kapha dominants can use this medicinal root to speed up their digestive and metabolic functions by drinking a glass of water boiled with slices of fresh ginger. This morning drink is a natural remedy to release mucus congestion in the throat and esophagus and also aids bowel movements.

Ingredients for the Kapha-Decreasing Morning Drink: 2.5 deciliters (1 cup) water and 1 teaspoon grated or sliced ginger

Preparation: Boil the water with the sliced ginger in a pan for three minutes. Pour the ginger water into a glass and stir with a spoon before drinking. Drink at a moderate temperature.

A Short Yoga Program in the Morning

After finishing the kapha-stabilizing drink in the morning, practice a short yoga program for kapha. This can lighten the mind, strengthen the body to support the circulatory and respiratory systems, and tone the heart, lungs, and blood vessels. You can learn more about yoga therapy for kapha in chapter 18.

Go for a Walk

There is no better way for kapha dominants to start the day than to go for a walk in the morning. The solid nature of kapha needs to move around as much as possible. Since kapha dominants generally love nature, they should try to spend some time every day close to the water, earth, or woods. Though all physical movements decrease kapha, walking is one of the best exercises to incorporate into the daily routine and to practice at all ages and in all seasons. A morning walk refreshes the mind and relieves heavy feelings in the heart.

Change Your Patterns

People with kapha prakruti have difficulty starting new disciplines and making transitions from old to new habits. Like the takeoff of an airplane, they might need a lot of energy to lift away from their present routines, but if they make the effort on the runway, the rest of the journey will be lighter and take them to higher levels.

With the right planning, we can change our daily routines without affecting our normal schedule too much. For instance, we could take the stairs instead of the escalator, or leave home a little earlier in the morning and walk to work. (If your workplace is not within walking distance, then park your car a short distance away or use public transport and get off a few stations early to get your walk for the day.) Remember that if you want to implement any discipline in your life, you need to find only one reason to do so. (But if you don't want to, then there are hundreds of excuses.)

Early to Bed

There is a tendency among kapha dominants to stay awake late at night and wake up too late in the morning. This routine is harmful to their health since it increases kapha and leads to symptoms related to an earth-water imbalance. To maintain a pattern of sleep, Ayurveda recommends that kapha dominants go to bed at 10:00 p.m. and wake up at 5:00 a.m. If you are a kapha dominant, you also need to make sure that you are not sleeping more than eight hours at night and not taking a nap during the day.

Daily Routines to Stabilize Pitta

Wake Up Early and Enjoy the Morning

Feeling energetic in the morning and tired in the evening is a common pattern for pitta dominants. They are alert at the beginning of the day and continue to be enthusiastic through the middle of the day, but their energy drops drastically in the evening.

Use the morning energy to make the beginning of the day pleasant and positive. Ayurveda recommends physical exercises such as yoga asanas and mental exercises like meditation as additions to the morning routine to maintain the harmony of the pitta force. Apart from yoga, other activities where the body and mind interact in a meditative way, such as walking, swimming, or gardening, can be good options to balance the fire and water elements in the system. If you are a pitta dominant, remind yourself to exercise not because you dislike your body but because you love your body.

Pitta dominants need to be extra cautious in direct sunlight (especially if living close to the equator and during hot summer days) since their skin is sensitive to heat. To take advantage of the healing rays of the sun, wake up early and let the morning rays shine on your skin and into your eyes (without looking directly at the sun). If you live far from the equator, make sure to get at least a few minutes of light on your body every day, which is important for the optimal function of your systems.

Practise Yoga to Stabilize Pitta

Disciplined practice of a pitta-balancing yoga program can regulate the fire and water elements in the body and mind systems. Yoga therapy can soothe the mind, release tension from the muscles, support the function of the digestive system, and tone the liver, pancreas, and small intestines. On the yoga mat, keep in mind that you are practicing your individual program to relax and connect with your body and mind, not to compete or to prove anything to anyone. You can learn more about yoga therapy for pitta in chapter 18.

Drink Enough Water during the Day

Pitta prakruti is warm in the body, and compared to the other two dominants, this body type needs more water to cool down the system. Because of the excess movements and the high performance of the central heating system, pitta dominants lose more water through sweat, especially during the seasons when the outside temperature is high. How much water a person needs to drink depends on their level of physical activity and the amount of water their body loses during the day. It is essential to drink an adequate amount of water to maintain proper blood circulation, which supports the function of the white blood cells that protect the body from pathogens.

Avoid Overheating the Body in Direct Sunlight

Ayurveda recommends that people with pitta prakruti avoid overexposure to sunlight, especially at midday in the summer, since they have sensitive skin and a higher chance of getting sunburn and heat-related symptoms from the direct rays of the sun.

Changing the lifestyle according to the seasons and the time of day is essential for everybody. For instance, if you are a pitta dominant (prakruti or vikruti), summer is the hottest season and noon is the time of day when you need to be extra careful with your physical and mental activities. Since the strength of the sun changes according to how close you are to the equator, you can feel the intensity of heat in your body and change your activities accordingly. If you don't take the climate factor into account, then when the temperature outside is high, the fire and water elements aggravate the force of pitta and release the stored water in the body as sweat, leading to dehydration and increasing the risk of skin diseases.

Take a Break (or Even a Short Nap)

As we have learned, pitta dominants have high energy in the morning and less energy in the evening, a pattern that is often magnified by their active lifestyle. A brief nap at noon can restore the energy and extend the enthusiasm until the evening. If you are in your office or traveling and can't take a proper nap, then just take a catnap, sitting relaxed with closed eyes for a few minutes, breathing in a relaxed manner, with a mind free of thoughts (or at least with fewer thoughts), as if you were almost asleep. (Should you choose to lie down after lunch, make sure you have taken a short, slow walk after eating your food in order to support your digestive system.)

Cool Down with More Water

For a pitta dominant, there is no better company than water, and swimming is one of the best ways to spend time with this healing companion, especially on warm summer days. During the hot season, take showers in the middle of the day to reduce excess heat from the largest organ of your body, the skin, which will help control the force of pitta.

To reduce stress and relax the muscles, pitta dominants can lie in a bathtub for fifteen to twenty minutes in the evening before bedtime. If the mind is still turbulent with multiple thoughts hindering relaxation, listen to some calming instrumental music and synchronize your breathing with the rhythm of the music.

Steam baths are part of many general health regimens, but if your pitta is aggravated, you need to make sure you are sitting or standing in a steam room where your head is outside the sauna and only your body feels the heat. (In an aggravated state of pitta, avoid all kinds of saunas where your head is inside the steam room. Overheating the head can affect the brain coordination and the sensory receptors of vision, hearing, smell, and taste.)

Slow Down Your Body and Mind

Since the pitta force often releases excess energy from the body and mind, generating intense actions and thoughts, Ayurveda recommends that pitta dominants take occasional breaks in between projects to keep their energy level steady throughout the day. Because of the intense focus of the pitta nature, if they engage in a particular task for a long time, they might feel pressure over the eyes (or even get headaches) as a sign to take a break. In this state, instead of pushing the body and mind to continue to work, it is recommended to go for a slow walk or stretch the body and take deep breaths to relieve the tension in the muscles.

This helps to relax the system and regain fresh energy to continue with the tasks for the rest of the day.

Don't Skip a Meal

For a pitta dominant, digestion is a gift if the stomach is fed at the right time with the right food, but it can be a curse if the person does not maintain a daily food discipline, skipping meals now and then. Compared to the other two dominants, pitta has the most powerful digestive system and the highest levels of digestive acids and enzymes; hence, not eating on time can lead to pitta-related health issues. When the secreted acid in the digestive system does not encounter food to break down, it can irritate the lining of the stomach and intestines and cause ulcers and tumors in the long run. Since pitta dominants are at risk for issues related to hyperacidity, they need to eat on time and choose the right food for their digestive system.

Be Flexible to Reduce Stress

People with pitta prakruti are firm in their beliefs. They don't compromise easily, which makes them the most stressful characters in different situations in their daily life. If you are a pitta dominant or have excess pitta in your system, understanding your own characteristics and the characteristics of the people you interact with in your community, at work, and in your family life is the first step to handle various life situations without the pressure of stress. To make it even better, try to slow down and listen to other people's ideas and find ways to cooperate with them without losing the core ideas of your projects and plans. This flexibility in attitude can help you improve your leadership qualities and excel in all fields, as you recognize the fact that the people you are involved with in your life have different qualities and characteristics according to their PDE, their presently dominating elements.

Allow Yourself the Gift of Sleep

Quality sleep can cleanse the mind-body system and restore the energy for the following day. For pitta dominants, the sleep train arrives early in the evening, and they need to go to bed around 9:30 p.m. to catch the train for a good night's sleep. From now on, see this evening fatigue as a gift rather than something you have to fight against.

Daily Routines to Stabilize Vata

Early Morning Sleep for Vata

This sounds contradictory to many health regimens that suggest waking up early in the morning to get a fresh start to the day. But for a typical vata dominant, this theory does not apply, since they need kapha energy to maintain their health, which they can gain by eating kapha-increasing food and sleeping during the kapha time in the early morning.

Traditional Ayurveda recommends that vata dominants sleep a little longer in the morning to improve the immune power of the body and the stability of the mind. Since most people can't stay in bed in the morning on weekdays, I suggest getting a long morning sleep on the weekends, especially in situations where the force of vata is disturbing your system, generating anxiety or other uneasy feelings.

Open Your Eyes to the Garden of Peace

When you wake up in the morning, stay in bed for a few minutes and invite nourishing thoughts, colorful butterflies, to the garden of your mind. During those first minutes of your day, encourage your mind to choose thoughts filled with inspiring ideas and exciting plans about what you are looking forward to experiencing in the coming hours of the day, or over the weekend, or even in the years ahead.

Have a Spiced Drink on an Empty Stomach

To support the digestive system and clean the esophagus and stomach by eliminating the gases formed in the digestive channels during the night, drink a glass of vata-balancing spiced tea on an empty stomach in the morning.

Ingredients for the Vata-Stabilizing Morning Drink: 2.5 deciliters (1 cup) water, 1 teaspoon grated or sliced ginger, half a lime, two cardamom seeds, two pieces of clove, a pinch of fennel, and a small cinnamon stick

Preparation: Boil the water in a pan with the ginger, cardamom, clove, fennel, and cinnamon for three minutes. Strain the water into a glass, squeeze the lime juice into the glass, stir with a spoon, and drink at a moderate temperature.

Nourish Your Natural Talents

The most successful people in the world are the ones who have found their natural, inborn talents and made their passion into their profession. Although people with vata prakruti have artistic abilities in their core nature, because of a lack of discipline and self-confidence, most of them stay hidden. On a base level, the vata nature is unorganized and scattered, which makes it hard for this prakruti to adjust to mainstream life in a family or society. If you are a vata nature by birth, instead of seeing these characteristics as limitations to progress, see them as the raw material needed to be successful as an artist, and use these artistic qualities in your work. For instance, if you are struggling with your vata characteristics, and your mind is drawn to painting or writing, use your scattered thoughts and unsettled feelings as the base of the theme you are going to write about in a journal or paint on a canvas. Here, painting or writing is not just artistic work, but is self-healing therapy for the artist.

Whether you are a talented singer or sculptor, or gifted with any other talent, explore your inborn gifts and nourish them. Otherwise, they will stay in the back of your consciousness and disturb your mind throughout your life. These disturbances often manifest in the mind as fear, anxiety, or other uncomfortable feelings. One could say that vata dominants often get pregnant in their heart with creative ideas, and if they neglect to nourish these ideas and don't give birth to the creation, these feelings create an emotional ebb and flow inside their mind.

Establish a Routine in Your Life

Start your search for your inner potential by trying different creative activities until you find your inborn talent, and once you find it, practice it every day with discipline. For instance, if you realize that you have an interest in writing, then write a few pages every day. If you have trouble getting started, try to spend at least half an hour daily in front of your writing table and jot down (or type) whatever comes to mind. When you practice your writing or other talents as part of your daily morning (or evening) routine, your trouble in getting started will disappear and your gifted talents will naturally flow from your heart.

Even though vata prakrutis are born with unique talents, many of them do not reach their potential in their desired field because of a lack of discipline. But once they believe in their talent and understand that it is the key to their success, they can establish a habit and make it a part of their daily life. To make the inborn talent a profession, vata dominants should invest some time in finding their passion and nourishing it every day. There is nothing better in life than making your passion into your profession. The day you succeed in making your talent into your profession is the day your holiday begins. Then you never work again in your entire life; instead, you do something you love.

Stay Warm as Much as Possible

One of the general characteristics of vata is cold. And if you are a vata dominant (by birth or because of an imbalance in the air and ether elements), this is what you need to concern yourself with most of the time. Not everybody can live in a country close to the equator all year around and get the natural warmth of the sun. But as a vata type, if you understand this part of your nature, you can at least make your living area (your house and office space) warm, or choose clothes that keep you warm and comfortable during the cold seasons. Also, always choose warm drinks and food rich in spices, which will comfort you like a warm blanket inside your stomach.

Choose a Serene Environment

Vata dominants have a vibrant energy and a tendency to get involved with similar people and environments. This can make for more turbulence in their life, since the vata mind often holds a mixture of fear and excitement, and is attracted to people and situations that stimulate these sensations. For the sake of creativity, you can expose yourself to these kinds of situations, but most times in life choose a peaceful environment in which to calm and ground yourself. When your mind is steady, you focus better on your utmost creativity, and with a disciplined practice you can climb the ladder of success step-by-step.

Do One Thing at a Time

Mindfulness is an important lifestyle practice to stabilize vata. Since the force of vata is formed by air and ether, the domination of these elements makes the mind scattered, with multiple thoughts and feelings. For instance, a vata dominant can be enthusiastic and cheerful one moment, but anxious and negative the next. Vata dominants often have several ideas and plans for their life, which can make it hard for the mind to come to conclusions. This creates confusion and frustration in the later development of their thoughts. If you can recognize the influence of vata in your mind, you can work on reducing the intensity of the force by doing one thing at a time. Bring your maximum focus to the moment of action until it is over. (You can practice mindfulness not just in your work but in every action, whether you are chewing your food or sipping your tea.)

Establish a Regular Eating Schedule

Difficult digestion (vishakha agni) is one of the major health issues caused by the aggravation of the vata force, resulting in gas and stomach-bloating symptoms. Since the level of agni, the digestive fire, is low in a vata-dominated digestive system, it is necessary to add the right spices to the food to aid the digestion. Also, eating warm food and eating small amounts but at regular intervals are ways for vata dominants to improve health and immunity. You can follow the vata-stabilizing food recommendations in the previous part of the book.

Avoid Heavy Exercise

Every exercise program should be designed according to a person's health condition. If vata is the dominant force, practice light exercises to maintain stamina for a longer period. Heavy exercise in a state of excess vata can not only cause damage to the bones, muscles, and ligaments but also lead to inflammation and pain in the body, as well as make you feel mentally drained. Practice yoga therapy to stabilize vata with grounding asanas and meditation exercises, which you can find later in this book.

Set a Fixed Bedtime

Considering the role of high-quality sleep in maintaining optimal health and immune power, try to get a good night's rest, especially if your body and mind are dominated by the force of vata. Compared to the other two dominants, vata has difficulty getting quality sleep since the depth and length of sleep can vary from time to time and from season to season. In old age, vata increases and disturbs the sleep, and it has a considerable effect on people who are born with vata prakruti. The habit of staying awake late at night makes vata dominants more fatigued the next day and can lead to sleeping disorders at a later stage. As a solution, even on nights when you do not feel tired, try to be in bed at a fixed time, since even just lying down gives your body and mind a rest.

General Daily Routine Recommendations to Stabilize the Three Forces

Kapha

- Wake up early
- Stay active during the day
- Vary your routines
- Seek out new experiences
- Avoid sleeping during the day
- Try not to accumulate material possessions
- Go to bed early

Pitta

- Enjoy the mornings
- Avoid excessive heat
- Balance rest and activity
- Don't skip meals

- Drink plenty of water
- Don't overwork
- Try to be flexible

Vata

- Wake up slowly
- Avoid strenuous and frantic activities
- Choose serene environments
- Maintain regular habits
- Do one thing at the time
- Get enough rest
- Stay warm
- Go to bed on time

Chapter 14

SLEEP FOR RECOVERY AND OPTIMAL IMMUNITY

Sleep plays a major role in maintaining the immune power of the body. Missing a few hours of sleep in the night can slow down the functions of the immune system and make the body more prone to catch a cold or flu. In this chapter we will study the sleeping tendencies of different dominations and the guidelines for optimal rest, including sleeping hours, sleeping positions, and pre-sleep preparations.

Sleep plays an important part in a person's health, especially in maintaining the natural immunity of the body. During sleep, with the force of vata, old body cells are destroyed and discharged from the body, and with the force of kapha they are replaced with new cells. When the toxins are eliminated properly, the force of pitta can maintain an uninterrupted function of the immune system and thus preserve a disease-free body. Considering the fact that cell replacement and toxin elimination play a major role in supporting optimal health, we can understand the importance of sleep.

During sleep, a wide range of immune-supporting cells are enhanced, like macrophages, B cells, T cells, mast cells, the endothelial cells that line the interior of the blood vessels and lymphatic vessels, and different stromal cells that support the connective tissue and produce cytokines—a cell protein responsible for the immune signals that are necessary to control and destroy infected cells in the body. A lack of quality sleep, however, can weaken these immune-supporting cells and thus the resistance power of our system. If a person gets very little sleep, like less than four hours a night, it can also increase the risk of heart-related problems and diabetes. Lack of sleep can lead to low levels of cytokines proteins and antibodies that are necessary to fight against infections.

The amount of sleep required to maintain a healthy immune system differs from person to person, and children need more sleep than adults. People with wounds or illness also require more hours of sleep to support the body for the healing process. While an adult needs around eight hours of sleep each night, a teenager needs nine to ten hours of sleep to maintain a natural level of immunity.

Ayurveda emphasizes the need for quality sleep for each domination by giving sleep recommendations according to the PDE (the presently dominating elements) of a person. If we adjust the sleep hours and patterns according to the PDE, we can balance the elements in the mind-body system and maintain a good resistance power at all ages and in all seasons of life. Let's take a look at the following chart, which explains the sleeping patterns of different mind-body types and how much sleep a person needs to maintain good health according to their PDE.

Sleep Patterns and Requirements of the Three Forces

The Corresponding Force of the PDE (Presently Dominating Elements)	Energy Level in the Morning	Sleep Quality	Sleep Patterns	Average Sleeping Hours	Optimal Sleeping Hours
Kapha	Difficult to wake up	Sound sleep—hard to wake up	Stays up late at night—tends to sleep during the day	Eight hours or more	Seven hours
Pitta	Energetic	Light sleep—tendency to wake up during the night but easily falls asleep again	Regular—warm, sweating, and restless some nights	Seven hours	Eight hours
Vata	Easy to wake up but tired during the first hour of the morning	Light sleep—often wakes up during the night and has difficulty falling asleep again	Irregular—often has strange dreams	Six hours or less	Eight hours

Sleep Therapy

Everyone goes through periods of sleeping issues in their life. But insomnia is becoming a common problem in our society because of our modern lifestyle, which encourages late-night activities. Nowadays, since many people can't get their natural sleep and rest, their bodies can't maintain the potential resistance power. To a certain extent, we can solve our sleeping problems by maintaining a discipline of going to bed on time and lying down, even if sleep does not come as a natural blessing. By keeping this discipline, we tune our body and mind to a timetable, and eventually we will be able to catch the sleep train closer to our bedtime. Remember that sleep is a vital factor in maintaining immunity in the body, since some functions of the immune system can only be restored during sleep. For instance, while you are asleep, your body cells produce cytokines and restore the resistance power, maintaining these immune-supporting proteins in the system.

To improve your body posture and breathing while you are in bed, choose your sleeping position according to your PDE. Choose savasana (corpse pose) for kapha and sayana balasana (sleeping child pose) for vata. Pitta dominants can choose either of these two positions. For them, the most important thing is to sit in vajrasana (diamond pose) before sleeping in order to calm the mind and relax the muscles of the shoulders, face, and lumbar region, which might have been tense during the day.

Savasana for Kapha Dominants

People dominated by the earth and water elements often suffer from congestion in the respiratory channels. If you are a kapha dominant, lie on your bed on your back in savasana (corpse pose) to prepare your body for sleep. While going to sleep, this pose helps to achieve a maximum level of oxygen flow in the lungs and gives the utmost rest for all the body's systems. This posture also promotes good blood circulation and better function of the lungs.

Vajrasana for Pitta Dominants

We often get caught up in the comforts of our modern lifestyle, which weakens our muscles and makes our body less flexible. For instance, the chairs we sit on during the day are made to promote comfort rather than strengthen the muscles of the body. If we look at the rural villages in some of the more economically developing countries of the world, we can see that people are sitting on their haunches, whether they are working, waiting for a bus, or using their flat toilets on the ground. These natural sitting practices give strength to the spine and muscles, even in older ages. But if we look at the more industrially developed countries, people are using comfortable chairs, sitting and working long hours in their office, where they spend one-third of their lifetime, and are having problems with stiffness in the shoulders and neck. If you spend most of your working time in front of a computer or looking at your phone, the condition can be even worse. Although these are general problems in our modern world, I have seen the worst cases among pitta dominant clients, since their muscles easily get tensed in these kinds of working environments. People with pitta prakruti can fall asleep quickly, but muscle stiffness and related pain can disturb their sleep during the night.

To prepare for sleep, sit on your bed with your legs bent underneath you in vajrasana (diamond pose). Let your palms rest on your thighs or knees, and gently inhale and exhale a few times until you feel your mind settling into a state of peace and your body into relaxation. If you have difficulty folding your knees in diamond position, place a pillow in between your calves and the backs of the thighs. (If sitting in vajrasana is difficult for you, sit on a meditation cushion or a chair besides the bed.) After taking a few relaxing breaths, lie down on your left side. Place a pillow between your inner thighs, and if you are still feeling some trace of stress from the day, hold another pillow close to your chest while preparing for a good night's sleep. (While getting ready for sleep, make the room fresh by opening the ventilation or window to create enough air circulation inside.)

Sayana Balasana for Vata Dominants

For a vata dominant, anxiety is one of the biggest mind-related issues, and this feeling can be high in the late evening before bedtime. For this reason, traditional Ayurveda suggests that vata dominants not go to bed lying on their back, facing the ceiling, which aggravates the vata force and thus the level of anxiety. Instead, lie on the stomach, half bending one leg and arm out to the side to get a close contact of the heart region (chest) to the bed, which invites a grounding feeling. This is sayana balasana, which literally means "sleeping child pose." Placing a heavy blanket over the body, especially over the legs and hips, can also improve the quality of sleep. (An illustration of sayana balasana can be found on my website at https://janeshvaidya.com/ayurveda/vata/.)

To reduce vata and improve the quality of sleep, drink a glass of warm plant-based milk boiled with cardamom and saffron. This evening drink from the traditional Ayurveda recipes can help vata dominants achieve a grounded feeling and thus better sleep during the night.

Recommendations for Better Sleep

In a well-balanced state of elements, all dominants can adapt any sleeping posture according to their comfort. However, because of our modern working style and improper beds, many of us are getting neck pain (in the cervical region) or back pain (in the lumbar region) and stiffness or inflammation between the shoulder blades (in the dorsal region), disturbing our natural sleep.

Make sure your bed provides the support you need. In ancient India, yogis slept on wooden planks, which was one of the secrets behind their powerful bodies. In traditional Ayurveda centers in the villages in India, they recommend that patients sleep on cots made of medicinal wood, such as neem or kino wood. The wood for a patient's cot is chosen by the Vaidya, according to the type of disease to be treated.

To regain the natural strength of your body, avoid soft beds for sleeping. Even though a hard bed can give you muscle pain in the beginning, see it as an exercise pain, and in a few weeks, notice how your muscles are getting stronger by adjusting to the hard surface. (Lying on a hard surface is not recommended for people who suffer from arthritis.)

The quality of your sleep also depends on how you arrange your bedroom, adapting it for a good night's sleep. Try not to use any electronic equipment in your bedroom. Electronics with magnetic fields or devices that transmit or receive signals from outside, such as mobile phones, can disturb your brain during the night. If you do have any electronic devices in your bedroom, make sure they are at least two meters (six and a half feet) away from your head.

While pitta dominants should make the bedroom cool and airy by adjusting the ventilation, vata dominants should keep the bed warm enough with heavy blankets. Kapha dominants are naturally gifted with heavy sleep, and they have to make sure they get up from the bed as soon as the alarm goes off in the morning and open the curtains to let in the daylight to reduce the risk of falling back to sleep. (In countries where the mornings are dark for most of the year, switch on the bedroom lights to make waking up easier.)

Part 4
MEDITATION—
YOUR MIND MEDICATION

Our mind is a set of momentary thoughts and feelings that determine the level of satisfaction and joy in every aspect of our life. Our happiness or sadness is not dependent on what we own or do not own, but on what we think and feel. And if we can't control or decide what we want to think, then we can't fulfill our dreams. Instead, we live like a slave to our own thoughts and feelings for the rest of our life.

The most dangerous viruses stay in our mind, interrupting our life with unwanted thoughts and feelings. These mental viruses might have entered our brain during the early years of our life, from a difficult childhood or a difficult relationship during our youth, or later through our interactions with the surrounding society. Even though those people and situations have gone away with the flow of time, the viruses they spread to our mind stay inside our system and grow with us, bothering our present life from time to time.

We have all had some hardships in our lives, and most of us honestly believe that we have overcome the pain caused by those difficult situations from our past. But from my experience of working with clients around the world, I have noticed that most of us are not free from the pain and shame caused by the events during the years of our growth. Though our conscious mind tries to forget those incidents, our subconscious mind is constantly alerted by the viruses that entered through those wounds. While most of us suppress the difficult memories and continue to live as if nothing happened to our heart, some people go to therapy to find solutions to heal those wounds. Both of these methods work to a certain degree, but not completely.

Since ancient times, meditation has been considered a natural medication and a self-healing therapy for the mind, which can be practiced to clear the mind permanently of the past viruses. In this section of the book, I introduce the best part of the meditation I practice myself with the support of my ancestors' wisdom, which has helped me to overcome sorrows from my childhood. The meditations have helped me understand not only the meaning of everything that happened in my early years of life, but also how those experiences played a role in melting my heart and shaping me into the person I am right now.

We all have something in our past to heal, fulfill, and forgive. May these meditation methods help you, too, to achieve your goals and fulfill your dreams in the future.

Chapter 15

YOUR MIND IS THE ARCHITECT OF YOUR LIFE

In this chapter I will introduce the influential factors of the mind that shape our core personality and create our relationship with the outer world and, moreover, with our own life. Considering that our attitude is the outfit of our mind, it also affects the other people we meet in our personal and professional lives. Then in the next chapter, I will present traditional mind techniques that you can use in your daily practice to free your mind from the most difficult patterns you may face in your relationships.

Our health and immunity depend not only on what we eat physically but also on what we take in as our mental food and how we process it in our mental body. Considering that the functions of our body and mind are interlaced, whatever happens in one will affect the other. So if any thoughts or feelings create a negative energy in our mind, it will affect the health of our body by obstructing the normal function of our systems and thus challenge our natural immune power.

Like the adage "An idle mind is the devil's workshop," if we don't feed our mind with organic food—and by that I mean creative and inspiring thoughts—our mind will be occupied by unhealthy, pessimistic thoughts: poisonous food that creates uneasy feelings inside. Many people believe that positivity is a natural feeling and we don't need to work to create it in our daily life, but that instead, positivity will come into our mind when the time is right or when everything works well in our life. But considering the amount of negativity that exists in our world, we need to train our mind every day and develop the capacity to absorb the positive energy from every situation. Otherwise, if we don't feed our mind in time, then like a hungry horse, our mind will go out and pick its food on its own, and most probably find it from the rubbish pile: bits of negativity that other people have thrown out, waste that can poison our mental body. When we understand this, we can make it a habit to practice some mind techniques every day to achieve the mental immunity we need to resist any kind of negativity trying to invade our mind and create disease in our mental system.

Considering the fact that thousands of thoughts pass through a human mind every day, ask yourself this question: Among your daily thoughts, how many are actually uplifting? It is good to remind ourselves that our mind is the architect of our life. Our thoughts are the starting point of our every action, and each of our actions is a cornerstone of our health and wellness, so we can understand what we are actually doing to our life by processing stressful, anxious, and depressed thoughts in our brain.

We all know that if we thought we had a choice, we wouldn't choose the thoughts that give us an uneasy feeling in our mind, which means we wouldn't select a thought that makes us stressed, anxious, or sad. But most times we feel like our thoughts are not a conscious choice. This happens when we don't have a good connection with our inner world; or, to put it another way, we lose control of our mind when our consciousness lives only in the outer world.

The way to get back into our inner world and take the lead of our mind is to practice meditation, which can help us connect with our true self and understand ourselves, our abilities and limitations, on a deeper level. And once we understand ourselves, it is possible to understand other people in our lives as well, and establish better relationships with them by building bridges of communication between our hearts.

Meditation is the medication of the mind. Regular practice of this ancient mind exercise will help you rejuvenate your mind by cleansing it of the daily toxic thoughts and feelings that accumulate in the brain cells. In our busy lives, we often forget to cultivate the most important seeds of thoughts that can grow into fruitful feelings. Whatever we earn in our life, whomever we meet on our path, at the end of every evening, we can return to our own mind and contemplate the overall feelings from our experiences that day. By understanding and forgiving our mistakes, and clearing out any feelings of sadness, guilt, or anxiety, we can prime our mind for a good night's sleep and prepare for another journey at the next dawn. When we wake up the following morning with fresh thoughts, once again searching for new experiences, we continue to walk through the same streets, but with more energetic and positive feelings in mind.

Understanding Yourself and Others

With the wisdom of Ayurveda, you can understand other people on a deeper level, which helps to establish a better relationship with a person's heart. But first, before trying to understand the other person, understand yourself better by knowing and accepting all your sides. While some of your characteristics might have been evident from birth, others you developed through the life situations you have experienced. That means that, according to Ayurveda, all the physical features and mental qualities you've had since the beginning of your life are characteristics of your dominating force at the time of your birth, and are considered your core personality. And when you spend a lot of time with someone, you need to understand your own as well as the other person's core personality, which helps to avoid conflicts and disappointments between the two of you.

For example, suppose that your birth dominating force is pitta, and you are living with a partner who also has a pitta domination. Since the core characteristics of pitta are intense, adventurous, and intellectual, in a state of balance you both feel strong and passionate in your relationship. But during times of imbalance in the fire and water elements, the aggravated pitta shows the symptoms of stress and anger, and the two of you become dominating and argumentative, closing off all the good sides of your core personalities, which creates conflict in the relationship.

Problems can arise in all relationships, and can vary depending on what forces the couple have as their birth dominant one as well as their current state of disorder. If two people in a relationship are dominated by the same force, or have different birth dominant forces (for example, one person is dominated by kapha and the other person pitta, or one kapha and the other vata, or any other combination), then in a stable state they show the good qualities of their core personalities and grow together in the relationship. But in an unstable state, they show the symptoms of their aggravated forces, which undermines their mutual connection and all the positive sides of the relationship. Therefore, to establish a good relationship with another person, whether it is a relationship in your personal life or in your professional life, it is important to know the core personality, the birth dominating force, of the other person and yourself, and to understand the effect that the imbalanced elements and their associated forces can have on a person's behavior.

A fundamental problem in this world is (and has always been) a lack of understanding between humans. It leads to conflicts among families, disputes in society, and wars between countries. As we discussed earlier, if we know the core personality of each person in our life, and understand the behavioral science behind the different personality types, we can handle the humans in our society in a much better way and avoid getting upset or feeling angry in response to their unexpected behavior at different times and in various situations. Instead, we can observe them patiently, understand the functional force behind each personality, and act or react accordingly.

If my clients tell me that they hate their boss because nothing is working efficiently in their office, I can reply sincerely that I had already assumed that was the case. When they ask me how I could possibly know this about the situation in their office even before they told me, to their bewilderment I continue my explanation of the characteristics of their boss whom I have never met. They wonder how I could possibly know all this. The answer is that my knowledge is based on the simple mathematics of Ayurveda: if my client is a pitta dominant, with a vikruti in that force, and is working under a person who is kapha dominant (perhaps even with a kapha vikruti), it's no wonder that my client gets frustrated by the boss's slow way of making decisions and failure to efficiently implement them in the office. What I suggest in this situation is to understand and focus on the good qualities of both forces and learn from them by inspiring each other instead of clashing. This can help both personalities grow in their fields and work in a peaceful and nourishing environment.

We live in a society where we have to interact with different kinds of people in all areas of life, which means that if you know the general characteristics of each person, you can make your life easier. Imagine that you are going to have a party for your friends at your home and you know that some of your friends are kapha dominants, some pitta dominants, and some vata dominants. With this awareness, you know their strengths and weaknesses, and you know who is more punctual and who has problems with keeping promises. Now suppose that you want everybody present for your party by 6:00 p.m. Since you know that pitta dominants are normally punctual, you ask them to be at your place at the right time. But since the kapha dominants are laid-back in their basic character, you tell them to arrive at 5:30 p.m., knowing they will probably be late and arrive around 6:00 p.m. Since your vata-dominated friends are quite artistic and have a hard time keeping to a schedule, you call them the same day to remind them about the party and prepare yourself not to get upset if they don't turn up on time or don't show up at all. Here you can see how, with the help of Ayurveda, you can handle a situation better by getting to know the distinct personalities of the people in your life.

Considering the fact that we live in a society made up of different personalities, in order to become successful in our personal and professional lives, we need to practice the art of handling the minds of other people skillfully. To interact with all kinds of people in our life and deal with their behavior effectively, we need to learn techniques to understand and lead the mind through a path of light instead of darkness— not only the minds of other people who appear on our life path but also our own mind on our own life journey. Whether you are a leader or an entrepreneur, or merely a human who wants to be successful in all areas of life, you need to learn the basic techniques of directing your mind.

To learn the art of directing the mind, so that it gallops like an obedient horse on the track, you need to practice with your own mind, with the utmost discipline and patience. In the following chapter, you will learn two of the main meditation techniques to calm down and find peace within that I often share with my clients. These mind practices can help you focus in your work and be present in your personal life, without the disturbances of your usual stressful thoughts and feelings.

MEDITATION FOR YOUR
MENTAL IMMUNE POWER

In this chapter I will give you two kinds of mental practice. While the first one is a tool to scan your mind to find the virtual viruses that often disturb your inner world and generate different mental problems in your daily life, the second meditation technique is useful to defuse those harmful viruses by reprogramming your mind with joyful and peaceful feelings supported by affirmative thoughts. You will also find guidelines to set up your meditation practice according to your dominating force, which is controlled by your PDE, your presently dominating elements.

················

Meditation is a disciplined practice of the mind, and once you achieve a meditative mind through focused and continuous practice, you can deal with the difficult situations in your day-to-day life, keeping a steady and calm mental state by handling your thoughts and feelings in a mature way.

The major challenge you will face during your practice is the reaction from your own mind, and you can overcome the initial challenges only through determination and understanding of these inner conflicts. During your practice, you may feel like you are repairing a sinking ship in the middle of the ocean while standing in the same ship, your mind. But once you repair your mind, you can continue the voyage, enjoying the rest of the adventure along the never-ending waves of the ocean, your life.

During your practice, consider your meditation as a journey, a mental journey on the wings of your imagination. If you are a beginner to this mind practice, remember that everything that obstructs your imagination or judges your creative mind can be a hurdle and bring your mind back into the same hole of restless thoughts. During your practice, if you analyze your mind's behavior based on your scientific views, it can be an obstacle to dive deep into the practice of meditation. I suspect that some of my students will probably never be able to meditate, either because of their difficulty imagining something they can't understand with their five senses or because they have trouble changing their belief from who they *think* they are right now to who they *really* are in their inner world. This will stop them from attaining a spiritual experience in this life.

As the first step of meditation, I suggest that you practice patience and try not to be overambitious at any time in your *sadhana*, your practice, as this will only leave you disappointed and make it more challenging for you to enter a peaceful state of mind. The only thing you need to do right now is to kindle your imagination by practicing the following meditation techniques with joy and hope in your mind.

Svadhyaya (Self-Study)

In our modern educational system, we train our mind by learning everything from the outside, while in the ancient Vedic studies, every individual educated their mind through introspective work and used the outer world only as a canvas onto which to project the information that they gained from their inner world. This meant that every individual did their part to shape the world by contributing their unique talents from their mind to their society, while we in the modern world are compelled to shape our mind to plug our life into the existing system of the world without considering our real talents. Because of our modern educational system, most of the talents are not getting the opportunity to perform in front of the world, and thus many people live with dissatisfaction and disappointment in life, without knowing the real meaning of their life on this planet.

Most people in the world are confused about their inner talents, which are hidden until they are practiced and performed during a lifetime. And many people are leaving this planet without finding their genuine qualities. They live their entire life listening to the external voices, following the footprints of the people who walked before them, and believing in everything that they have learned from the outside world, but forgetting to listen at least for a few seconds to their own voice, scared to follow their own heart's desires. If they would have done so, at least one time in their life, that might have planted the seed of another belief in their mind and they could have lived a different life, a life of ultimate satisfaction, joy, and peace.

Remember, you are not dead and you have not lost the chance to enjoy life to the fullest, like millions of people before you. Take a deep breath and know that you are still alive, that you have enough time to make a radical change in your thoughts and beliefs, your attitude, and the rest of your life. The only thing you need to do right now is to step out from the procession of society, where everyone walks with the same kind of goal, the same wish, which is not personal, not your goal or wish. Once you are out of the line, you will see everything clearly. You will know what you really want and what you don't want. You will know exactly how you want to feel and live this life. There you will recognize the source of your uneasy thoughts and feelings that are creating the stress and anxiety to achieve something meaningless on this planet, which was once the fuel of your overambitious mind and society's formula to be a successful human. From now on, you will know that it was an external force that invaded your system from the early years of your life and became a dictator of your mind. And you will know that it is time to return to a state of mind where peace and joy exist, without the dichotomy of gaining or losing, owing or holding, but of being as you are in your inner world.

Mental Viruses

I agree that no mind can change overnight, considering the fact that a person's beliefs are rooted in their past. We were all born a child with a blank memory, which is like the hard drive of a new computer. As we pass through different stages of life, from our childhood to youth to middle age and old age, just like the hard drive of a computer, our memory stores millions of programs that have become our beliefs in life. While some beliefs nourish our life, some of them prevent our mind from growing further. Even similar kinds of beliefs can have the opposite effect in different people's lives. For instance, if a person believes in the presence of God in their life, and lives an honest life as a result of that belief, then that belief is helping the person develop good qualities and habits in life. Another person can believe in the same God, but because of their blind belief that God exists only in their religion and the only way to God is through the practice of the rituals of their religion, the person can become a fanatic and be disrespectful to people of other religions and religious practices. While the first belief about God is nourishing that person's good qualities, the same belief is nourishing the second person's bad qualities and restricting their mental development.

Whether the views are personal, social, political, or religious, or on any other aspect of life, it is good to remember that our overall life results from a set of beliefs that are planted in our mind over the years; and as long as we grow, like a banyan tree, the roots of our beliefs will spread out and go deeper into the unknown layers of the earth. What we see as our outside physical body is like the leaves and branches of the tree, but the core of the tree, our deep beliefs, is nourished through the roots that are invisible and hidden under the earth.

Through the practice of meditation, you can scan your mind and understand the roots of your thoughts and beliefs, and monitor if there is any belief that has been lingering in your mind for a long time as a virus, obstructing your mental growth. But even though you can sometimes recognize your viruses, it is not as easy to clean your brain as it is to clean your computer's hard drive. Once you have found your viruses, use the next exercise, the mind vaccination technique, which will help prevent further viruses from infecting your mind during the creation of thoughts and feelings.

To bring these methods into your life, we will begin with the first Svadhyaya practice, a mind-scanning meditation. Once you find the viruses in your mind, you can move on to the second practice, the vaccination technique. While the first practice helps you find the root causes of your mind issues, the second practice helps you defuse those virus programs with new antivirus programs in your mind.

Mind-Scanning Meditation

You are the result of your past, and to understand yourself deeper, you need to understand your past and how you reached this point in your life.

Preparation:

- Choose a day with enough time to be on your own.
- Bring a notebook and pen and, if needed, a cushion to sit on and a shawl to wrap around you.
- Find a quiet place in your house or in nature, and sit in your preferred meditation pose.
- Find your posture and spend a few minutes observing the current state of your mind and body.
- Imagine that your mind is a house with two levels. The first level is the living area, where you usually stay, and the basement level is the cellar, where you store your old memories. Imagine there are twenty-one steps leading down to the cellar from the first level of your house. With this picture in mind, you are ready to start the mind-scanning meditation.

Instructions:

1. Breathe gently, inhaling and exhaling, and imagine that you are standing on the first floor at the top of the staircase leading down to the cellar.
2. Imagine that you walk slowly down the stairs to the cellar—the subconscious part of your mind—one step at a time, in

tune with your breathing. Each time you inhale and exhale, take one step down, silently counting backward from twenty-one to zero. The next step will be twenty, the next nineteen, and so on, until you reach the basement on zero. This breathing exercise, combined with the reverse count, is a self-hypnotizing method used to bring your mind into your inner world and prepare your consciousness for meditation.

3. When you reach the basement, search for the very first memory of your life. You may, for example, have a vague idea about some images or events from the early stages of your childhood. Think about those memories and try to add more images around them. Recall the faces and the places that influenced you during the very early years of your life. A tip is to start with some memories from the age of two or three, and study those images as if you were watching a movie in a theater. For instance, recall some images of your home where you used to play or where you learned to walk, or see if you can remember your favorite toys, clothes, or colors.

4. Move through your growing period, from your childhood to your youth to your current age, recalling scenes from each age. Observe your growth as if you were the main character in a movie developing with the story. For instance, see your first school days, classmates, teachers, and some events from those years. Or reminisce about your likes and dislikes, your hobbies, and your favorite music, movies, fashion styles, and idols during your teenage years. Then try to recall the days when you finished your education and left home, searching for a job, finding a love relationship, etc.

5. Once you have finished recalling your old memories, slowly walk up from the cellar to the first floor—the conscious part of your mind—taking the steps one by one with the count of your breath. Each time you inhale and exhale, take one step up, silently counting the first step as one, then the next

step as two, and the next as three, until you reach the first floor on the count of twenty-one.

6. Sit for a while with your eyes closed, becoming aware of the sounds around you and the feel of the air against your skin, giving your mind time to land in the present.

7. Slowly open your eyes and write down eleven happy memories and eleven sad memories from your life that you recalled during your meditation.

Later, read the happy and sad moments and think about how those events affected you to shape your present personality. See the indirect influence of those sad memories in your present life. If any of those incidents are bothering you in your present life (consciously or subconsciously), mark them as virus programs still running inside your brain and prepare for the next stage: clearing those negative programs from your mind.

Mind Vaccination Technique

This technique is a continuation of the previous exercise, the mind-scanning meditation. However, I suggest that you allow at least a few hours, or even a day, to pass before you do the second technique.

Preparation:

- Choose a day with enough time to be on your own.
- Bring a pen and the notebook you used for the mind-scanning meditation and, if needed, a cushion to sit on and a shawl to wrap around you.
- Find a quiet place in your house or in nature and sit in your preferred meditation pose.
- Use the meditation technique you are most familiar with to prepare yourself for the coming exercise. (You will find meditation guidelines later in this chapter.) I suggest you spend at least fifteen minutes in meditation before continuing with the following instructions.

Instructions:

Open your notebook and read through your list of the eleven happy and eleven sad memories that you wrote down after the mind-scanning meditation.

Take the saddest incidents from your past and think about the opposite feelings of those incidents. For instance, if you had a difficult childhood, or if you are still holding onto a memory of a sad event that happened in the early years of your life, think about what could be better if you'd had a chance to change those incidents. Try to see it as a puzzle where you can use your brain to change the behavior of the people involved, the mood of the situation, etc.

Now, as you are rewriting the drama that once was your life, you are free to change everything according to what you want, not according to your memory. For each sad incident in your life, write down your actual memory and then write your wish of how you would like it to have been. By practicing this puzzle, you can see that all the past characters are like puppets on your fingers and that you control the situation.

Remember that we all have some sad experiences from our past that exist only in our memory. But we still indirectly react to those incidents when we meet or think about people from those times and when we encounter similar situations. As an example, during mind development sessions, I often meet clients who are holding feelings of anger toward their parents. Those feelings from their childhood have grown in their mind through the years. I advise them to look at their parents as their children and see their actions from that point of view. By changing their point of view, this simple vaccination technique gives them relief from their negative thoughts when they interact with their parents.

With a calm mind, observe the saddest memories of your life and open them one by one for a detailed study. Believe that whatever happened is only in the past, and the most important thing in your present life is that you are still alive on this planet.

Should you need to, you can spend some time in meditation between each memory to anchor yourself in the moment.

The use of the mind vaccination is simple. With this technique, you recall a sad incident, and by finding a positive aspect of that situation (by looking at it from another point of view), you inject the new aspect into your mind. With this meditation technique, you can change the situation and the behavior of the people involved according to what you would have liked to have happened, instead of what you have stored as your memories. The reason we have this drama in our inner world is because we can't change our past, but if we let those sad memories stay in our mind, they can have a negative affect on our present and our future.

It is your duty to rescue your mind from the sad memories. When a sad memory enters your mind, tell yourself the following:

1. It is all in my past. If I defuse those memories, none of the incidents will affect my present or future life.

2. Whatever happened, I don't see myself as a victim. Instead, I see the difficult experiences and situations of my past as necessary steps to my present life.

3. Those incidents were the biggest lessons in my life, which not only gave me sadness but also gave my mind an invisible strength.

At the end of your practice, sit with your eyes closed and observe your body and your breath. Release any tension that has accumulated in the body with your exhalations, and let your mind rest by allowing thoughts to come and go without clinging to them.

Remember that you don't need to go through the whole mind vaccination process at once. Take time to get familiar with the exercises and acquaint yourself with your inner nature step-by-step. It is important that you feel you are in a safe space while practicing meditation.

Try to stay with your peaceful mind after meditating by avoiding outside stimuli from television, computer, or mobile devices for at least thirty minutes, or longer if necessary.

Meditation Guidelines for the Three Forces

Meditation, in its most basic form, is a disciplined mental practice to achieve awareness of our inner world, our thoughts, feelings, and emotions. Even though our mind is the chief practitioner in this exercise, we need to train our body to cope with this mental practice. That means we should prepare our body so that we can dive deep into our mind and start our inner journey. I suggest that you follow the guidelines given here with a few specific recommendations for your dominating force, which is controlled by your PDE (the presently dominating elements) in your mind-body system. You will find further instructions on how to tune your body and mind in the next two chapters on Ayurveda yoga therapy.

Take a Seat

When you meditate, I suggest that you sit with crossed legs in what we call *siddhasana* (or a variation such as sukhasana or padmasana). Sit on a pillow if needed. The most important thing is to sit with your hips higher than your knees. If needed, place pillows under your knees as well. If it is too difficult for you to sit cross-legged on the floor or on a cushion, you can sit on a chair. (It is important that you keep an upright posture while meditating, so try to avoid slumping in a sofa or comfy chair.)

1. Sit on the floor with your legs straight out in front of you.
2. Bend your left knee and bring your left heel close to your body, placing it by your groin area.
3. Bend your right knee and move it toward the front of the left ankle.
4. You can choose to leave your feet where they are right now, or lift your right foot and place it on top of your left ankle. In that case, bring your right heel close to your groin area. Slide the toes of your right foot into the space between the left calf and thigh.
5. Place your hands on each knee, palms up or down, according to the instructions for kapha, pitta, and vata later in the chapter.

Remember to alternate the position of the legs from day to day to avoid creating uneven movement patterns in the knees and hips. That means, for example, that if your right leg is on top one day, then put the left leg on top the next day.

Regardless of the sitting position you choose, make sure to keep a good length in your spine, keeping in mind that you want to maintain a natural arch of the spine, neither slouching nor overarching. The posture should be active but not rigid. If needed to maintain length in the back of your neck, you can tuck your chin in slightly.

Let your eyes gently close. Keep your face relaxed by softening the muscles around your eyes and ears. Release any tension in the jaw by applying a gentle smile to your lips. Make sure you are not clenching your teeth or pressing your tongue against the palate of your mouth.

I recommend that you breathe through your nose while meditating, as it will keep the breath steady and the mind focused.

Choose an Anchor

When you sit down to meditate, it is likely that you will encounter different disturbances from your body and mind. This is natural and nothing you need to worry about nor try to fight against or struggle to ignore. To help yourself sit through the physical and mental distractions, I suggest that you choose a symbolic anchor that will center you and bring your attention back to the moment. You can choose one of the following anchors or find your own:

- Your breath
- Sounds around you
- The sensations in your hands/palms

And So It Begins

Find a space where you can sit without being disturbed. Spend some time getting into the sitting position that best matches your physical state.

Scan your body to make sure you have found the proper alignment, and allow yourself to let go of any tension in your body and mind. Acknowledge your current physical and mental state without judgment.

Gently draw your attention to your chosen anchor, or, if you prefer, choose one of the sets of meditation guidelines described here for the three forces of kapha, pitta, or vata, depending on your PDE.

Meditation Guidelines for Kapha

Posture: To counter the tendency to slouch, a person with a kapha domination needs to put extra focus on maintaining a strong and upright sitting position. A cushion, stool, or chair can give you a lift if you have a tendency to slump forward.

Mudra: Choose a hand position that promotes mental clarity and energizes you physically, preferably with the palms facing up. Place your hands on your knees, with the arms active and the chest broad and slightly lifted. Fold the index fingers so they create circles, with the tip of each index finger touching the base of the thumb. Lengthen the other three fingers as much as possible without straining the muscles of the hand.

Meditation Technique: With each inhalation, lift your body up and lengthen your spine. Imagine a line of energy from the base of your spine to the crown of your head. Keep this sensation of lightness on the exhalation. This will help you stay alert through your meditation.

Meditation Guidelines for Pitta

Posture: For pitta dominants, especially if pitta is in a state of excess, there are two areas of the body that need extra care at the beginning of a meditation session: the shoulders and the solar plexus. Before taking your seat, lie on the floor for a few moments, with your palms resting gently on your belly, just above the navel. Let the touch of the hands melt away any stress or feelings of constriction in the solar plexus area. When you feel ready, slowly find your way up to your preferred sitting position, keeping the softness in your torso. Place your hands on your knees and move your focus to your shoulder area. With an exhalation, release any tension around the shoulders, neck, and shoulder blades.

Mudra: As a pitta dominant, you can choose to place your hands on your knees with the palms facing up or down. I recommend that you pick the option that puts the least amount of strain on your shoulders. Let the tip of each index finger touch the tip of the thumb, forming a circle. Soften the muscles in your palms and fingers, and allow that relaxation to spread along your arms to your shoulders.

Meditation Technique: With this meditation technique, I want to encourage you to soften your focus as well as your ambition. This is an opportunity for your competitive mind to relax. Remind yourself that there is nothing you need to achieve in this moment. Allow yourself to follow the steps below by merely observing the sensation of your breath.

Throughout the session, let your breath flow in a natural rhythm, without trying to control it. The rhythm of the breath can change from day to day or even during a session. Observe these changes without judging or criticizing.

The first times you try this meditation technique, I suggest that you stay with the first practice, step 1. After a few sessions, you can add the next step to your practice, and so on. However, always stay with each step for a few breaths before continuing.

1. Become aware of the breath as it enters and exits through your nostrils.
2. Expand your awareness to the nasal passages.
3. While still being aware of the air entering and exiting through the nostrils and the nasal passages, experience the sensation of the air as it reaches the back of your throat and the windpipe.
4. Follow the flow of the air as it enters through the nostrils and flows through the nasal passages and the windpipe, filling the lungs and then leaving the lungs, to return through the windpipe and exit through the nostrils.

During your practice, if you notice that you are feeling stressed or agitated, make a mental note of the feeling and then continue with your practice.

Meditation Guidelines for Vata

Posture: For people with excess vata, I recommend using a chair only if absolutely needed, as sitting on the floor will make you more grounded and stable. Put on enough clothes to keep you warm, and wrap a shawl or blanket around your hips if meditating in a chilly atmosphere.

Mudra: Place your hands on your knees, with the palms facing down. Form a circle with each thumb and index finger by letting the tip of the index finger touch the tip of the thumb.

Meditation Technique: Start your meditation session by inviting your mind to land in your body. Ground yourself by becoming aware of the areas where your body is touching the ground. With each exhalation, direct the energy flow toward your pelvic region, making your posture stable and secure. Each time you inhale, make sure that a rooted feeling keeps you connected with your secure seat, both physically and mentally.

To further balance the air and ether elements that control the force of vata, we can add a mantra to the meditation practice.

Mantra Option One:

Listen to the sound of your breath. When you breathe in, you will hear the sound "So," and when you breathe out, you will hear "Ham."

Mantra Option Two:

With each inhalation, actively say the word "So," and with each exhalation, say "Ham." You can say the words out loud or just feel the vibration inside as you form the sounds with your mind.

The "So-Ham" mantra leads the practitioner to peace and better concentration. It often translates as "I am that," but you might understand it more deeply if you imagine that while breathing in, you fill yourself with life energy ("So"), and while breathing out, you release your ego and your limitations ("Ham").

Easing Out

Meditation is a flight lifting your mind from the ground of your daily life to reach new heights. When your spirit ascends, you feel lighter, and like a bird in the sky, you glide without obstacles. But the takeoff from the runway, the initial preparation of the flight, is the hardest part of this mind practice for many people who are not used to flying. And it is even harder for people who don't believe they can fly.

To make your dream journey come true, trust in your flight and be on the runway with your continuous meditation practice, preparing for takeoff. For some people, it can take a few weeks or even many months to lift their heavy mind from the ground, to leave behind their sorrows and stress and reach above the clouds, losing the gravity of their reality, which they realize is incomplete and unreal once they reach the space where they move gently like a bird.

And every time you return, remember that you are flying back into turbulence, landing in the mundane world with all it entails. So take it easy every time you return to this world. Take a few deep breaths and relax before you open your eyes. When your meditation session is over, I suggest that you spend a few minutes in savasana (recommended for kapha and pitta) or sayana balasana (recommended for vata) to give yourself time to readjust to the world around you.

Part 5
YOGA—
YOUR PERSONAL THERAPY

If you don't open up your house or ride your bicycle for a long time, they won't function after a while. Just as an abandoned house accumulates fungus on its structure or an unused bicycle becomes rusty in its mechanical parts, our body also develops problems in the absence of proper care and regular attention.

As I explained earlier, our body is made up of trillions of cells, and each cell contains five elements: earth, water, fire, air, and ether. These fundamental elements control our body's functions, including the production, growth, and death of cells with the actions of the three forces—kapha, pitta, and vata, respectively. While the earth and water elements generate the force of kapha and support the generation of cells, the fire and water elements generate the force of pitta and maintain the cells' health. Meanwhile, to make space for new cells, the force of vata, formed by the air and ether elements, destroys the old cells and expels dead cells through the excretory channels.

If any of the three forces gets aggravated by an imbalance of the corresponding elements, the overactive force disturbs the natural rhythm of our internal system. For instance, if the earth and water elements are out of balance, they aggravate their associated force of kapha and thus store more fat in the cells than they actually need, which leads to obesity and water accumulation in the tissues. While the extra weight becomes a burden for the circulatory system, the excess water increases the risk of generating inflammation that invites pathogens into the system. In the later stages, obesity can lead to cardiac issues, and inflammation becomes the cornerstone of many diseases, potentially threatening our life. Similar to the problems with excess kapha, if there is an aggravation in the pitta or vata force, our body shows its irritation as symptoms or, in the long run, as disease. While an excess of pitta generates problems in the digestion and metabolism, aggravated vata destroys more cells in the body and makes the aging process faster than normal.

Our body is an incredible mechanism, and like any mechanism, our internal systems need maintenance and daily care to stay disease-free and functional in all seasons and at all ages of life. Otherwise, like an unused bicycle, our systems will get rigid and immobile through the years, and our structural elements imbalanced and our forces aggravated, destroying our system and speeding up the aging process. If we continue to neglect to provide essential services to our system, then just like an abandoned house, our body will be fertile ground for harmful external microorganisms.

As our own personal bicycle, our body needs movement, and like our house, our systems need timely cleaning and maintenance to remain functional for our entire life. Yoga therapy is one of the great tools of Ayurveda to keep our body and mind systems in better shape and support the immune system by stimulating the lymphatic system, conditioning the lungs, and maintaining a good flow of oxygenated blood to the organs. But remember, yoga is not merely a set of asanas; it is a physical, mental, and a spiritual journey through your life.

THE FIVE PILLARS OF YOGA

In the next chapter you will learn more about how to create a personalized yoga therapy program according to your PDE, the presently dominating elements in your mind-body system. But first, in this chapter you will learn about Ayurveda yoga therapy and the role of its five stages in the therapeutic practice of this ancient wisdom. In Sanskrit, the five stages are known as dharana, pranayama, vinyasa, asana, and dhyana. With these five pillars of yoga, the practitioner becomes their own therapist, building the base of their daily yoga program to practice solo at all ages of life.

· · · · · · · · · · · · ·

Dharana

Always make sure to start your yoga practice with the right *dharana* (focus). The purpose of this initial practice of your yoga program is to set your body and mind to be focused, to direct your attention from the external affairs of your daily life to the moment of practice. Sitting in a comfortable position (preferably vajrasana), let your mind drift into the present moment. Set an intention for your practice according to the energy you wish to create in your practice. In the next chapter you will learn the basic objectives behind the therapeutic practices to balance the fundamental elements and thus the corresponding forces in your body.

Pranayama

One of the primary tools of yoga is *pranayama*, or controlled breathing. Regular practice of this ancient exercise can vitalize the prana (life energy) that resides in the solar plexus region of your body. The solar plexus is the center of your inner galaxy and controls all of your body systems and mind functions. Through practicing pranayama, you can recharge your solar plexus and create a free flow of prana. According to the present state of the imbalances in your system, you can choose breathing techniques for the aggravated forces and return to a stable state by regulating, stimulating, or grounding the energy in your system. You will find introductions to basic breathing practices in the next chapter.

Vinyasa

A *vinyasa* is a sequence of movements connected with the breath to create a free flow of life energy. After restoring prana in your solar plexus region through the pranayama exercises, practice vinyasa to distribute your life energy to the cells of your body. In Ayurveda yoga therapy, the vinyasas are built to balance the PDE and regulate the five elements and the functions of the corresponding forces in the mind-body system.

Asana

An *asana* is a body posture that is steady and firm yet relaxed. Through the disciplined practice of asanas with concentration (dharana) and tuned breathing (pranayama), you can achieve flexibility, balance, and strength. Choose the asanas according to your PDE (presently dominant elements), your state of balance or imbalance, health or disease. In the next chapter you will find a short series of asanas for each of the three forces.

Dhyana

After the four previous practices, the practitioner comes into a natural state of awareness of their body, mind, and life energy and the connection between their inner and outer worlds. In this stage you will recognize your physical and mental pain. Since you released the tension in your muscles and joints through your asanas, you will also be more aware of your hidden feelings and emotions, such as fear, anxiety, suppressed anger, and sadness, which are starting to be released from the depth of your base chakras. That is why *dhyana* (reversed focus) is the last stage of your yoga therapy program. It helps you detach your mind from worries and anxieties. By drawing your focus away from your present thoughts, you will return to a state of bliss. Dhyana practice helps the further restoration of life energy in your solar plexus and its flow into the core of your body and mind even after your yoga practice.

YOGA FOR YOUR DOMINATING FORCE

In this chapter I will give you short yoga programs that help to balance the different dominating elements and their corresponding forces. You will also receive guidelines to set up your practice and tune your mind on the yoga mat. We will also look into the challenges you might face while practicing yoga. This will vary depending on the force dominating your system at the moment. As with any lifestyle practice, it is important to know your PDE to structure and tune your daily yoga practice.

· · · · · · · · · · · · ·

Yoga Therapy for Kapha

If your PDE is kapha, you need to maintain an interest and a routine in your daily yoga practice, which is one of the biggest challenges you will face. To get inspired to get onto your yoga mat, find a corner in your home for your practice where you can put your personal touch with your favorite colors and accents. Once you are on your yoga mat, try to keep your mind enthusiastic and explore your limits with your body postures. Throughout the practice, keep your mind focused and imagine a light feeling in your body. Since kapha is grounded and heavy in its basic characteristics, choose asanas that lift your body from the ground and promote upward movements. Practice each posture with determination and a feeling in your mind that this is both your therapy and a treat at the same time.

Yoga Therapy for Pitta

If your PDE is pitta, make sure to practice with ease, since pitta dominants have a tendency to do everything too perfectly, which will only generate stress and frustration at the beginning of your practice. If you are a pitta dominant, it is good to be aware of these tendencies and train your mind to be patient. And remember to avoid self-criticism at any stage of your practice. When you come to your yoga mat, see it as a space where your body can take rest and your mind can relax. Choose the asanas that can reduce agni in the solar plexus region and release tension from the muscles. It is important not only to choose calming asanas for your mind-body system but also to perform the asanas gently so that your body does not get hot and your mind does not get stressed during the practice. In other words, keep your body and mind cool throughout the yoga session. If you find at times that you can't relax, just lie down on the yoga mat until you feel totally relaxed, and then continue your practice.

Yoga Therapy for Vata

If your PDE is vata, the biggest challenge is to maintain the discipline to do yoga every day. To do that, the most important thing is to set your mind to practice by telling yourself something like, "I'm not sure about tomorrow, but today I am going to do my yoga." If you repeat this mantra every morning and bring your body to your yoga mat, convinced that this is only for today, you will get into a routine of practicing yoga every day without a break. If you are a vata dominant, choose grounding asanas that can release the tension in the lower abdomen area and the pelvic region. Throughout the practice, keep your energy level steady by performing the asanas gently, avoiding fast movements. Be in the moment and keep your mind calm and centered throughout the practice. Remind yourself often that you are taking good care of yourself with your practice, and never give up on your yoga, even during times of turbulence in your life.

Yoga Programs for Kapha, Pitta, and Vata

These following yoga programs are specifically designed to regain and maintain the body's natural flexibility, balance, and strength, considering the limited and often damaging physical movement patterns of our modern lifestyle. If we sit on comfortable chairs, walk with our feet locked into fashionable high heels, and sleep on soft beds, our joints and muscles will become stiff and sore and our posture crippled, and we will move like we are old even in our youth and middle age.

As our lifestyle patterns change, so do our movement patterns and the physical issues we face in our daily life. To address these issues, I suggest that you practice a personal yoga program (according to your PDE) in the morning to reset your posture and tune your energy for the day. In this section I provide three basic programs to choose from according to your PDE, one program each to stabilize kapha, pitta, and vata. If you are not familiar with the asanas, you will find the poses outlined on my website in the yoga therapy section.

If you need further assistance or a personalized program for a specific symptom or disease, I suggest that you contact an Ayurveda yoga therapist. If you are not able to find an Ayurveda yoga therapist in your area, you can refer to my book on Ayurveda yoga therapy and select the yoga asanas for your present health issues. By adding these extra asanas for your symptoms/diseases to your yoga program for your PDE, you will become your own therapist and can start practicing your individual program at home. The book also includes more than fifty Ayurveda yoga therapy programs for different symptoms/diseases.

Kapha Yoga Program

For a visual guide to this kapha yoga program, visit this page on my website: https://janeshvaidya.com/ayurveda/kapha/.

1. Dharana: 3 minutes
2. Energizing pranayama: 3 minutes
3. Mountain pose: 1 minute

4. Chair pose: 2 minutes

5. Downward dog pose: 1 minute

6. Plank pose: 1 minute

7. Downward dog pose: 1 minute

8. Seated twist (both sides): 1 minute + 1 minute

9. Upward plank pose: 1 minute

10. Savasana including dhyana: 5 minutes

Energizing Pranayama:

Lie down in savasana and place your arms in trident position. (If one or both hands are not touching the floor, place small pillows under both hands.) If needed, bend your knees, keeping your feet on the floor.

Inhale while expanding your chest to the sides, to the front, and to the back, visualizing that you are stretching the muscles between the ribs. Exhale while deliberately contracting the rib cage, squeezing all the air out of the lungs.

Pitta Yoga Program

For a visual guide to this pitta yoga program, visit this page on my website: https://janeshvaidya.com/ayurveda/pitta/.

1. Dharana: 5 minutes

2. Cooling pranayama: 3 minutes

3. Cat pose standing: 1 minute

4. Cat pose sitting: 1 minute

5. Downward dog pose: 30 seconds

6. Child pose: 1½ minutes

7. Crocodile pose: 3 minutes

8. Savasana including dhyana: 5 minutes

Soothing Pranayama:

Sit in vajrasana (diamond pose). Make sure you relax your face, jaw, neck, and shoulders. Place your palms over your solar plexus.

Inhale slowly, letting the lower ribs expand slightly. Exhale softly and let the lower ribs retreat. Focus on softening the diaphragm and calming and cooling the solar plexus area.

If you have difficulty sitting in a kneeling position, you can perform this exercise lying down on a mat on the floor.

Vata Yoga Program

For a visual guide to this vata yoga program, visit this page on my website: https://janeshvaidya.com/ayurveda/vata/.

1. Dharana: 3 minutes
2. Calming pranayama: 5 minutes
3. Mountain pose: 1 minute
4. Tree pose (both sides): 30 seconds + 30 seconds
5. Standing forward fold: 1 minute
6. Knees to chest pose: 1 minute
7. Sayana balasana including dhyana: 7 minutes

Lie down on your back in savasana.

On the inhale, imagine that you are filling the belly with air, and when you exhale, imagine that you are emptying all the air and let the belly sink. Inhale and exhale at even lengths.

MAKE A PROMISE

Gaining knowledge is important, but practicing that wisdom in your own life is the most important. Once you determine the health status of your body and mind with the help of Ayurveda, start your practice following the recommendations, and observe the results in the coming days. See every day as a brick with which you are going to build your dream fort, your maximum health and immunity, and patiently place those bricks one by one, day by day, with the right food, exercise, meditation, and yoga practices, using the information in this book. Make a promise to yourself at this moment that from now on, you will maintain discipline in your life, for the rest of your life, by using the natural tools of Ayurveda, and that you will live in a state of maximum health and immunity in all seasons and at all ages of your life by maintaining the correct balance of the elements in your mind-body system. And always keep the mantra in mind that happiness is your birthright and health is your conscious choice.

TALLYING YOUR TEST RESULTS

Key to TEST 1: Find Your Imbalance

If you answered yes to a question in the "Find Your Imbalance" test in chapter 5, circle the corresponding points in the following chart and tally them at the end.

Key to TEST 1: Find Your Imbalance

Question Number	Kapha	Pitta	Vata
1			1
2		1	
3			1
4		1	
5	1		
6		1	
7		2	
8		2	
9			1

Key to TEST 1: Find Your Imbalance (continued)

Question Number	Kapha	Pitta	Vata
10	1		
11	1		
12	1		
13			1
14		1	
15		3	
16		2	
17			1
18			1
19		2	
20			2
21		1	
22			2
23	1		
24	1		
25		1	
26	2		
27	2		
28	1		
29	2		
30	1		
31	3		
32			2
33			3

Key to TEST 1: Find Your Imbalance (continued)

Question Number	Kapha	Pitta	Vata
34		3	
35		3	
36	3		
37			3
38	3		
39	3		
40			1
41			2
42		1	
43	1		
44	1		
45	1		
46			1
47			1
48	1		
49			2
50			2
51			1
52			1
53		1	
54			2
55			1
56			1
57			1

Key to TEST 1: Find Your Imbalance (continued)

Question Number	Kapha	Pitta	Vata
58			2
59		1	
60		1	
61		1	
62		1	
63		1	
64	2		
65	1		
66	1		
67	2		
68		2	
69		2	
70		2	
71		2	
72		2	
73			2
74			3
75	3		
76			3
77	3		
78	3		
79	3		
80		3	
81		3	

Key to TEST 1: Find Your Imbalance (continued)

Question Number	Kapha	Pitta	Vata
82			3
83			3
84		3	
85	2		
86	3		
87		1	
88			3
89		3	
90			2
91		2	
Total number of points for each force			

Key to TEST 2: Find Your Core Nature

For each question in the "Find Your Core Nature" test in chapter 5, circle your answer (X, Y, or Z) in the following chart. At the end, tally how many items were selected in each column.

Key to TEST 2: Find Your Core Nature

Question Number	Kapha	Pitta	Vata
1	X	Y	Z
2	Y	X	Z
3	Y	Z	X
4	Z	X	Y

Key to TEST 2: Find Your Core Nature (continued)

Question Number	Kapha	Pitta	Vata
5	X	Y	Z
6	Y	X	Z
7	X	Y	Z
8	Z	Y	X
9	X	Y	Z
10	Y	Z	X
11	X	Y	Z
12	Z	X	Y
13	Z	Y	X
14	X	Y	Z
15	Z	X	Y
16	Z	Y	X
17	Z	X	Y
18	X	Y	Z
19	Z	Y	X
20	X	Y	Z
21	Y	Z	X
Total number circled for each force			

RECOMMENDED RESOURCES

For information about Janesh Vaidya and his work-life:
www.janeshvaidya.com

For further reading on Ayurveda: www.janeshvaidya.com/ayurveda

For more information on yoga therapy: www.janeshvaidya.com
/ayurveda/yoga-as-therapy

For reference books in other languages: www.janeshvaidya.com/books

For more information on Ayurveda and yoga therapy education:
www.janeshvaidya.com/ayurveda-education

For the author's latest blogs on Ayurveda in English:
www.janeshvaidya.com/english-blog

To Write to the Author

If you wish to contact the author or would like more information about this book, please write to the author in care of Llewellyn Worldwide Ltd. and we will forward your request. Both the author and the publisher appreciate hearing from you and learning of your enjoyment of this book and how it has helped you. Llewellyn Worldwide cannot guarantee that every letter written to the author can be answered, but all will be forwarded. Please write to:

Janesh Vaidya
℅ Llewellyn Worldwide
2143 Wooddale Drive
Woodbury, MN 55125-2989
Please enclose a self-addressed stamped envelope for reply,
or $1.00 to cover costs. If outside the U.S.A., enclose
an international postal reply coupon.

Many of Llewellyn's authors have websites with additional
information and resources. For more information,
please visit our website at http://www.llewellyn.com.